Saving your life one day at a time

seven ways to survive the modern world

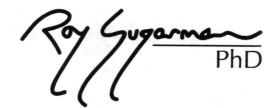

PhD

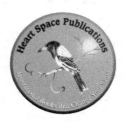

Heart Space Publications

Australia: +61 450 260 348

South Africa: +27 11 431 1274

www.graysonian.com

pat@graysonian.com

First printed in Australia in 2013

Copyright © 2013 Dr Roy Sugarman

Published in Australia by Heart Space Publication 2013

ISBN: 978-0-9872816-8-5

eBook ISBN: 978-0-9872816-7-8

Contents

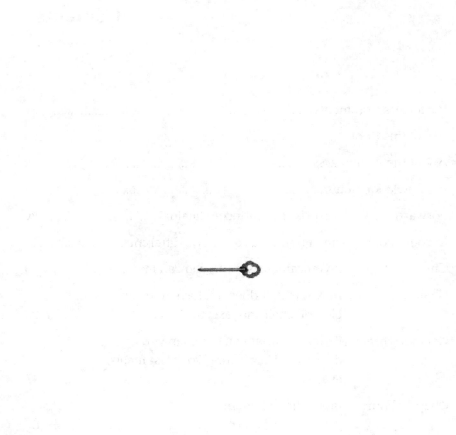

reviewers comments

"If the concept of beginning to 'rot' from the inside out doesn't motivate you to take on the challenge of living a fuller life, nothing will! Dr Sugarman delightfully blends humor, frankness and positive motivation to get you off that chair and fully living the life you were meant to live. With Dr Sugarman's coaching, you'll immediately understand the crisis while feeling fully empowered to reach the imperative of a healthier life now and into the future! Genius stuff!"
Dr Michelle Brennan-Cooke;
Vice president, Magellan Health Enterprises, USA

"Roy's seven ways are practical, doable, and life changing. This simple book, built from Roy's expansive research, is not just about surviving the modern world, it's about thriving in the modern world."
Scott Peltin,
Founder/Chief Performance Officer/Tignum and author of Sink, Float, or Swim

"*I found myself really getting inspired by it! It's incredible info and very readable. The rot starts early! Yikes! Got to get my ass moving!!!! Love it.*"
Yvonne Gomez,
ex-Olympian Skater, Olympic Skating Coach, NBC TV Director, and founder of GoGo Sport, San Francisco USA

"*Roy Sugarman hits the nail on the head with the Western lifestyle issues that are rotting us away. The take home message is that YOU hold the power for change on multiple levels. You have to read this book. Better yet, read it while standing up and moving about. Let's wrestle back control of our health from the environment. What say you?*"
Ryan Crandall,
Movement Specialist at Fitness and Yoga Integration, New Mexico

"*Dr Sugarman's brilliance is in the conversion of Applied Science into a totally practical, comprehensible approach for the everyday reader. He effectively solves life challenges for us with amazing clarity.*"
Ian O'Dwyer,
Functional Movement Expert and co-founder, PTA Global

"*It was with great enthusiasm that I read Dr Sugarman's new book. Roy's ability to create a "how to" for healthy modern living is immense. Making complex and involved topics easy to understand and apply is a skill that so few do well, and he has done that. Combining the science of vitality for body and brain, with a sure-fire recipe for achieving and maintaining it, separates this book from other authors that have tried this unsuccessfully. A fantastic read and a must for all ages.*"
Michael James,
Co-Owner, Primal Fitness: Sydney, Australia.

about this book

You know what to do but you never get around to doing it.

There is a ton of good advice out there, but you never take any of it.

Healthy lifestyles are something we aspire to every New Year, but never manage to accomplish during the year. New Year's resolutions have a short lifespan, and fail before February.

Where did our resolve go? Our energy gets used up by work and household duties and so there is not much left for family and fun. Every goal we set at work ignores the fact that we live for what we love, and that this love is invested in our lives at home, not work.

Although we get up each day and spend most of our time at work, for most people the workplace is filled with things we do not really care too much about, unlike our leisure time with family, friends, home, sport, hobbies, and holidays. These are the things we live for but our energy gets used up before we get home from work, leaving 70% of people tired from the day, with little energy to live life and love it after hours: 84% of people with depression are in the workplace if the American Psychological Association can be believed. Studies in Australia certainly indicate that this is so. We are all sleepwalking through life.

With mental illness and or chronic disease facing most people in their retirement years, there is little doubt that modern working life is not conducive to health and happiness during the working years, or after it. And although we know what we **should** be doing to have more energy for life, we seldom manage it. TV and newspapers tell us this every day.

The rot starts early: most kids and teenagers today are not getting enough sleep, are sitting hunched over a device for most of the day, are not exercising, and are eating things that should never be swallowed, let alone desired and nagged for!

In this book, peak performance expert Dr Sugarman shows you how to approach changing small but meaningful issues in seven areas of your life, which optimise your brain and body to the point where you can go home from work and still be able to enjoy what is really important to you. You will learn how to feel good and ready to live life longer, and love it.

In the meantime, doing these things will make you a more engaged and productive worker, and enhance your career. Translate these to your kids, and you will have happier and healthier children as well.

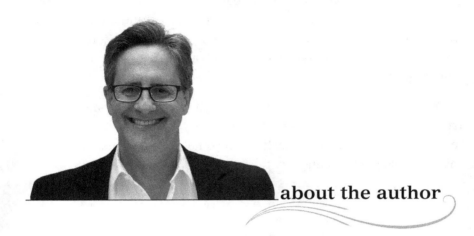

about the author

r Roy Sugarman is the Director of Applied Neuroscience at the world's premier athlete training facility, Athletes Performance and Core Performance in the USA and in that role is the current mindset coach for the US Soccer National Men's Team. He works with college and professional athletes, corporate executives and their staff, as well as personal trainers, coaches and Special Forces operatives, and a variety of clinical clients. Dr Sugarman learned early in his career that only an integrated combination of brain and body interventions succeeded in optimising our ability to get through the day at work, and still have enough energy in the tank to go home and enjoy what was most important to us – the people we love.

He trained and accredited in Clinical Psychology and Clinical Neuropsychology. With decades of experience in rehabilitation of severe traumatic brain and bodily injury, Dr Sugarman observed that integrating the science of both body and brain was essential to positive outcomes in healthy individuals as well. Working with damaged athletes, and then with healthy ones, he learned that most experts focus on only their medical speciality, ignoring the content of other specialists working with the patients, consequently neglecting most of the issues so important to a good outcome, or leaving them to someone else.

Gathering information usually studied in fragments across specialities, people have learned that body and brain are a single entity, and health in one, is health in the other: Dr Sugarman has spent his professional life doing just that.

Read more on **www.roysugarman.com**

acknowledgements

My mentors across nearly sixty years have been many, but most are now departed. I truly have been fortunate to stand on the shoulders of geniuses, and often studied beneath them. They taught me that the pinnacle of being a teacher is to see your students rise beyond you, and while many of my teachers have said the same of me, I can also say the same of those I have taught and treated across the decades. Associate Professor Les Koopowitz is still around, and my gratitude for his teaching and knowledge shared is enormous, as is the welcome Sue Leighton and the staff give me when I go to Adelaide. Dr David Manchester, my colleague in Motivational Interviewing and beer in Surrey Hills is a motivational genius.

It is not those that were kind or inspirational to me when I was young that matter as much now. It is those that I have around me now that mean so much.

My wife and my two daughters, who have followed me around the world, in some cases to their detriment, but I believe they have and will reap the benefits of living and dancing large. My sister, who has known suffering in her time and somehow keeps on going and inspires me to do the same. My cousin and business partner Brian, my in-laws Doreen and Ronnie who think I am a genius, but who still have not convinced my wife of that.

My colleagues Paul Taylor, Jeremy Howell, Yvonne Gomez, from USF. The brilliant Ian O'Dwyer at Noosa. My colleagues at Athletes Performance and Core Performance, the inspirational Mark Verstegen, Craig Friedman, Masa Sakihana, Sue Falsone, Amanda Carlson-Phillips, Danielle LaFata, Nick Winkelman, Nick Anthony, Dan Zieky, John Stemmerman, Dan Burns and so many others too numerous to mention there, but they know who they are. To Jesse at US Soccer and Amy at AP/CP who keep me in Nike and Adidas splendour for all seasons, and save me a fortune in sportswear. My athletes across the world, from the USA to Russia, for their inspiration and sacrifices. In particular, Tim Howard, Michael Bradley, Clint Dempsey, Sean Johnson, Josh Gatt and other US soccer stars who are just awesome and inspire me.

The people at Primal Fitness, who save my life one day at a time, Aaron and Kate Callaghan and Michael James, and Lachlan as well. Ian Stokol who built my website. These guys are in my life, do incredible things for me, and do it for nothing. Go figure.

And the staff from US Soccer. The wonderful Juergen Klinsmann and the coaches and players from the US National Men's team who are so inspiring in their willingness to integrate just anything that will take them higher and further.

And finally, my parents, Vicky and Stan, who understood that every day is a battle. One taught me to fight, the other to love, and I am still trying to work out which one works better.

Dr Roy Sugarman

Foreword:

the prism of enduring health

odern life is increasingly disabling and killing us and our children. This starts when you are young. We are perhaps the first generation who will outlive our children. Half the kids born in western societies since 2000 will become diabetic. They are already born with jaws that are too small, leading to crowding of their teeth. And smaller brains. More behaviour problems and more learning problems are emerging. Sunlight and the content of our stomachs or diet now show up in the literature on Autism, Multiple Sclerosis, and other chronic afflictions.

Our lives are lived in a world we have created, not the world we were created for.

As societies become more affluent, their health declines. As we make more money, and improve our quality of life, our health declines. Yes, it does. We are setting the stage of chronic disease as we move further away from the hunter-gatherer diet.

You know what happens when you shine a white light on a prism? It breaks up into a rainbow of seven colours, the visible spectrum. Red, Orange, Yellow, Green, Blue, Indigo, Violet.

Your enduring vitality is like that: shine a light on it, it breaks up into seven domains that need to be coloured in. This book attempts to do that for you, focusing a spotlight on each of the seven arenas you need to consider in achieving enough vitality, more energy to get through the day with more left in the tank, and then sleep peacefully. Most people do not get to do that, mostly because they live in a modern world for which increasingly the body was not designed, with ongoing damage to body and to brain.

What is enduring Vitality, or a term I prefer, building resilience? According to the originator of the term 'wellness', Dr Halbert Dunn, who lived and worked in the Fifties, this refers to an integrated method of functioning which is oriented toward maximizing the potential of which the individual is capable. It requires that the individual maintain a continuum of balance and purposeful direction within the environment where he or she lives. He also stated that wellness was a series of actions we take in progressing toward an ever-higher potential of functioning. All of this points to body and brain homeostasis as a lifetime goal.

So there are seven shades of the prism of enduring health, each one is simple enough and therefore, easy to achieve, without a large dedicated chunk of time that you do not have. Yes, there are indeed quick fixes, small things you can do that make a huge difference. Willpower is nothing, because when you get good at the detail, the big picture follows. Looking at the big picture, on the other hand, and how you have failed before, takes the wind out of your sails: do the small stuff well; the rest takes care of itself. Or you can rinse your mouth with sugar water to improve your willpower and stay away from the cookies.

Let me make one thing clear: I am no guru. Like Viktor Frankl, when I stand on the shoulders of a giant, I can see forever. What I have in this book is not much of what I have found, but what great people in the various domains of health have taught me. Hang around long enough in the presence of greatness, with good solid knowledge of body and brain behind you, you pick up what works and what does not, what is folklore and what is solid science, and more importantly, what the average person can readily incorporate into their daily life.

Let's face it: we all live on deficit time, and when we have time to 'relax' we do things that in the fullness of time will kill us: sitting, drinking, eating. Living a proactive prismatic life not only leads to a better outcome for us and our children, but for our daily working and home life today, now, not just sometime later, when it may be too late. Rewards are immediate. A monumental effort is not required. Small things you do now can make an immense difference, immediately and later too.

Just be brave enough to shine a bright light on the little things that change the future for you, from the threat of a miserable series of visits to the doctor, from moaning to your children about your aches and pains, to the joy of hearing people say WOW, you are so not 60/70/80!

You may be saying to yourself, look, I am healthy, but in reality, you may have started a process already that will lead you to suffer later on in life. That may deprive you of the future you always dreamed of. You may die at thirty-five, and just not realise it until you are sixty or seventy, when you first find out what has gone wrong. The rot starts early, silently, white-anting us and leaving little sign, so you need to start preserving your tomorrow, today.

Dr Roy Sugarman

Introduction:

small things make a huge difference

My Irish colleague Paul Taylor, a research professor at the University of San Francisco (with whom I co-presented in *Body and Brain Overhaul*, an eight-part TV series on Australian TV) and I agree: we are ancient bodies in a modern world, which is not a good look for most of us. This content of this book forms the basis of my rehabilitation work in laymen's terms, when I attempt to return damaged people to optimal life, to extricate them from the loneliness of their injured lives – in my terms.

By this I mean that virtually nothing that we do during an ordinary day is in sync with how our bodies were designed to work and heal. Compared to even our grandparents, we do not sleep the same hours, work the same hours, move in the same way, socialise, eat and drink, and so on. There is an endless list of things we now do, which we never used to do, and a host of things we never do, which we used to do (read that again if you got lost!). So we are increasingly less healthy, one generation at a time, which means all unhealthy hell is about to break loose for our children, and theirs in turn. X and Y generation is followed by…?

The upshot of this is that arthritis, mental illness – such as mood and anxiety disorders, diabetes, obesity, dementia, heart disease, and a host of other modern plagues such as cancer come to dominate most people's lives at some stage. This is not just when they are old, but striking earlier and earlier in our lives.

We live longer now, so what?

Instead of working hard and enjoying retirement as our ancestors do, we spend the last ten years of our longer lives in doctor's rooms and taking more pills, instead of on the family yacht. Sometimes, thanks to investing our money with the likes of Bernie Madoff, like musician Leonard Cohen's unfortunate manager, we have to carry on working until we drop as our 401k pension funds become worth nothing, and companies pay disability money to thirty to forty-year olds, who come from college with very little work ethic, while expecting to design an App and make a fortune from working at home. Great expectations, failed narcissism.

Page | 2

Disabling Lifestyles of the West:

It does not have to be this way. However, increasingly it is for most people, and not just the elderly. I am told by my colleagues at the Disability Management Employer's Coalition meetings that the thirty to forty-year-old worker in America is increasingly the biggest user of disability money in history, and they are still poisoning their kids with bad, processed food, so that they will be the first generation to outlive their kids. Diabetes? Obesity? The military in America is finding it hard to sustain its search for recruits who are healthy enough for service, and ejecting hundreds of unfit personnel a year.

So what on earth is wrong? Actually, the entire problem is our fault, not the world's, or the workplace, it's what WE do and what WE never do that is making younger and younger people seek disability, and makes growing old a miserable time for many. What we have done to our world, to what we eat, drink, absorb and breathe. These are the dangers you know, but do nothing about. The rot starts early as we spend more time sitting around and eating junk.

Death and disability are bred into our lifestyle. Our lifestyle is not conducive to health and happiness, or leading a productive home and work life, or raising healthy and happy children.

The experts worldwide that I talk to agree that our lifestyle is the single major cause of most modern malaises, at home and at work. A lifestyle that is out of sync with how our bodies and brains are built to function best, or what we are born with and then manage to ruin a good system along the way. And yet all we have to do is what visionary Jack Lalanne said from the 1940's on until his death at ninety-six years old: get off your asses and stop eating that c**p. It starts there, and it is that simple. This you know, this you ignore. Let's see if we can change that.

Deficit Time and convenience eating:

And here is the root of the problem: modern life is so deficient when it comes to spare time that we find it hard, perhaps impossible to factor in healthy behaviours into our busy, time-hungry lifestyles. Deficit time is the biggest excuse that people have for not living a healthy, productive life, exacerbated by the arrival of children.

There is a huge market for convenience food – food that has been interfered with so we can cook and eat it faster. There is a massive market for 'treat foods' and 'snacks, which are loaded with awful chemical concoctions, or with labels that lie about the hidden slow poisons inside. That is not good.

The world is full of electronic media that works best when we sit down. That is not good either. Thus there are two major 'bricks' in the wall; firstly, eating badly and secondly, both adults and children increasingly leading a sedentary existence.

We and our children do most of our brainwork sitting down. That is fatal in the long run, and while not immediately fatal, in time it causes a lot of suffering, earlier and earlier in human life as we spend more time on our butts and eating increasingly unhealthy junk, masquerading as food and drink. Whenever you walk in a room, people are polite enough to demand you sit down and be comfortable: why, do they hate you so much they want to kill you? Or should they encourage you to run on the spot and live life longer and love it?

Modern Lifestyle is the single greatest cause for most of the preventable illnesses plaguing us today.

That means the solution to multiple mental and physical illnesses is in our hands, not the doctor's. The heads of innovation at the big health insurers in the USA have all requested just one thing of innovators:

keep people away from the doctors. The doctor's pen, says the New York Times, has become the most expensive piece of equipment in medical costs in the USA. Especially when the pen writes the word: 'disabled'. This word should never be used in the context of You at any time of your life.

One of my friends at Harvard, Dr Marcia Scott, a doyen of the community and adviser to the American Psychiatric Association, has commented that if we could help primary care practitioners quantify the complaint of 'fatigue' in their patients; we could control the disability industry. So much about the advice around us is vague, it is hard for you to work with it and change yourself for the better. What should you do?

Aspiring to become healthy is not enough. It is like a New Year's Resolution. Although on January 1st I decide to change my eating, work-out, give up smoking and be happier, on January 2nd I still get up at 7a.m., get one child out of the door, take the second one to school, eat breakfast, shower, get me and the wife out the door, do stuff, race back home for a meeting, clean up, do the beds, washing, emails, post office, banking, dash to meetings, dash to pick up one kid, then the other, give them a meal, homework supervision, rush out to buy dinner stuff, cook, bring in washing, and on and on until bedtime, way too late, at 11:30 pm… Deficit time does not allow for lifestyle change to easily just happen.

My new year's resolutions turn out to be aspirations that simply find no time and space in my lifestyle. I tread water until holiday time, and go away on holiday and get sick. Most doctors in holiday destinations only take their break when the tourists are still at home: business is too good during the peak holiday season to consider taking vacation time then!

Increasingly, our socialization is done on social media, not face to face. We send harsh and nasty emails instead of talking on the phone or in person. The Bell Telephone company used to ask us to reach out and touch our family, no longer living near us. Now, it is worse. Skype allows us to be face to face with anyone, anywhere, but we cannot see their whole body, or hold them close. We increasingly lack empathy, an essential for close and sustaining friendships. Young girls use relational violence to drive their so-called friends to suicidal depression. Airbrushing has given way to Photoshopping to drive our girls to anorexia. Young men no longer slow dance close to a girl, so never learn about the sexy spot at the base of her spine, or the fragrance on areas she would like to be kissed.

We think we can achieve anything, and tell our children that, but we no longer understand how extrinsic reward systems have mutated to be intrinsic in the twenty-first century. How autonomy, mastery and purpose fail us in the modern world, and how little things do matter when money is off the table as an incentive.

We have spent our lives moaning to therapists about our misery, and taking pills that do not work in most of us, but few of us understand the power of Positive Psychology, or manage the three positive events to one negative daily event that must drive our motivation, or the five to one to drive our relationships. Alternatively, the eleven to one that drives our group forces is yet to be understood as a critical element by most.

We work like slaves to Mammon, but have no idea about healthy, proactive recovery.

Most of us, most of you, have no clue how to live life longer, protect our children from an early demise, or appreciate that we will not be around forever. What is your legacy? Are you now prepared to stop abusing your life and your children's lives? Or will you accept the good advice that you just will never take? Leaving them money to manage their disability is not exactly the legacy I have in mind for my kids.

This book shows how aspirations to be healthy can become small, cumulative goals, can fit into the busy work and leisure day, and can create substantial resilience for daily work and daily life, so that there is time and space to live life longer, loving it along the way. And allow us to go on holiday and NOT get sick!

Firstly, I will explain why measuring where you are now leads to better management. Secondly, I take you through six main arenas of your lifestyle where little things you change will make a huge difference. The first big two are movement and nutrition. And although I will be telling you things you may already know, the next chapter will tell you how to *actually accomplish* these two large bricks in the house of healthy – how to motivate yourself to get off your backside and stop eating that rubbish.

Then I follow up with another four arenas, in mindset terms as we call them, of social contact, managing your motivation, defending your body and brain against modern life, and creating happiness at work and positivity at home, with the new energy you have found. If life is a journey, do it in baby steps as I do not want you to get sore feet or trip up.

And think of the next generations. You will leave this world a sadder and less healthy place than your parents gave to you. What you take for granted as normal is not, and never was. It is getting worse, and it is your fault if you do nothing. All that is required for your children to suffer disability and death is for you to carry on doing what you are doing, a black, glacial existence. Money won't be enough to protect them from themselves.

Let us shine a light on that prism. We begin with Red – Becoming aware.

The term *Wellness*, or *Vitality*, or *Resilience* has been defined by the Singapore-based National Wellness Association as an active process of becoming aware of and making choices toward a more successful existence. So let us talk about becoming aware, so we can manage our vitality.

Chapter One

red
if you can measure it, you can manage it

*S*tan was a family man. A sportsman for his entire life, leading an active life with swimming and jogging, devoted to his family. He visited the doctor at fifty-five complaining that on his morning jog, he felt a little breathless – the first red flag. His doctor measured a few parameters, such as blood pressure and an echocardiogram and told Stan he would be lucky to live another two weeks. Stan made it to eighty-three. Never again did he spend more than a few months without measuring how his body was doing, and what he was doing to stay alive. Stan was lucky, keeping angina at bay until his five-way bypass at sixty-six, living on until eighty-three. Finally, an infection of his gall bladder killed him, and although he had stopped smoking at fifty-five, his blood vessels never recovered, so there was nothing to deliver nutrition to his organs at eighty-three, otherwise he would have lived on longer. His wife, who ignored the red flags, died suddenly at sixty-six, during her first cardiac investigation, an angiogram. These were my parents.

Each of the brain body optimisation areas in this book has a way to measure them.

When I head to my doctor, he chats a bit about annoying stuff, and then finally gets around to examining me: stethoscope, blood pressure, cardiac sticky bits on my chest, thermometer in my mouth, all the measuring gizmos he can get (including sticking his fingers where no-one is allowed). Then he sends my blood to be measured in a laboratory. Next, he tells me how to manage the things that are wrong, how to get my blood pressure under control, how to deal with cholesterol, and how many drugs to take: *then of course, I ignore him. Nevertheless, that is for later…*

Why are you not doing this measuring stuff? Chances are you have those measures available to you, just seconds away. Not for what the doctor alone might measure, but for the things you need to measure so you can manage the things that are killing your body, your brain, and your future happiness, and that of your children.

In essence, we start dying at thirty-five and finally realise it at seventy when things go brutally wrong. Then we are 'shocked'. "OMG, I am sick!" That was a long time coming; we just used the wrong measures or criteria to alert us to the looming disaster.

We need to manage this thing called lifestyle a lot better, and measuring it is where we start, so we know where to start. For us as well as our kids.

The point I am making here is that the **rot starts early**. You need to know the exact minute when it starts.

Why? Well, let us talk about genetics. Do not worry, I will not get technical. I do not understand most of it either, but we do not have to be geniuses to work with our genes.

Genes, like children, need a garden to play in, a place to switch on, and switch off. There are good genes and there are bad genes. Some will switch on, no matter what, like Huntington's, a fatal movement disorder, or Tay Sachs, a brain disorder, requiring both parents to contribute the gene. Some will need lifestyle to switch them on or off. What we do know is that tiny areas in our genetic structure respond to lifestyle and turn on little switches that nobody wants to see in the ON position. Lifestyle environment issues push those switches on or keep them off.

Genes that can be really nasty if they are turned on and are in reality being turned on by environmental factors, the things we do or do not do, and those that get done to us, a process called epigenetics. So if great-granddad had the same bad genes as you do, how is it he smoked, drank, and ate tons of fat and still lived to be eighty-six without a statin drug or a cholesterol test? How is it that despite the amazing drugs available today that we do not live longer than many of our ancestors? The answer is... Lifestyle. Measure how many miles great granddad walked. It turns out he did a marathon a week more than we do today. Not sitting on his butt in front of a computer or TV most of the day. It seems that he spent a lot less time in front of the wheel of his car. Turns out he and grandma did a ton of lifting, carrying, walking, and other good stuff. Monitor his food and it was mostly organic, mostly fresh, and sometimes home grown, some delivered, mostly from a local greengrocer who grew his own stuff. Measure what he drank and you will find his hydration was better because he mostly drank tap water or tea, and he took in less sugar, less salt, and less Omega 6 by eating fewer processed foods than you do. His grocery store was a short walk away, and sold very little else other than fresh food, canned stuff, and cigarettes. Measure his electricity and he used fewer and less power-consuming appliances, tumble driers, dishwashers, washing machines, vacuums, and he certainly did not sit in front of a computer or iPad. Nor spend time thumbing a smart phone. Even his phone book required some heavy lifting! A lot of the football he watched was in stadiums with limited seating, so he stood. He climbed stairs, not elevators, or travelators or escalators. As a child he ran outside, in parks, on his bicycle, skates or pedal car, swam, climbed to the top of jungle gyms and slides, now banned because of silly litigation issues. Families had one radio, so they gathered round, reading and stimulating their minds, close to one another, and the single fireplace or stove, on which all meals were cooked from scratch. His milk was whole milk, his spread was butter, and it was full fat. Vegetables came in all colours, and were fertilized with stuff that never saw a factory and which we will not talk about in polite company, but it stank. He mowed his lawn with a manual machine and he painted the house himself, and did the wallpaper. During the war, he used his bicycle. He drank limited alcohol, mixed with water, not sugary 'alcopops'. His washing machine was a big sink outside with a bar of soap that stank of carbolic. He polished his shoes with a brush, not a wipe on and dry. On a nice day, he and his wife went for a walk with the dog. A dog, who he washed, by hand, after he watered the garden, by hand, where he worked on the weekends to grow his vegetables, which he fertilized with nitrogen from his own body when he had had too much to drink, or from the nightsoil.

They often got sick, to which the one to two kilograms of bacteria in, and on their bodies responded with a good immune system and fought it off. Antibiotics were unknown for most of their childhood, during which only the strong survived. There were no antibiotics in the Sunday roast, and the cows and lambs they ate had eaten grass, not grain, or sheep brains or fish.

They ran to the telephone, ran to the bus, hung up the washing, turned the Xerox machine by hand, ironed, cycled or walked to the store, paddled their canoe, promenaded by the beach, and so on. They did not see all the world's dramas on TV five seconds after it happened, never stressed by the disasters affecting millions over TV at dinner. During the war, they went hungry for long periods of time, which helped lengthen their lifespan. They learned to not worry about things they could not control, and seldom saw other people nude or envied their bodies. News was limited to the radio, to a channel or two, or to the pace of reading a newspaper slowly on the train. Another country took three weeks to sail to. People died at home, not in a ward, penetrated by steel and plastic and chemistry.

At work, they carved, cut, sewed, punched, pulled, lifted... you get the idea? They lived and experienced a different life. And with the same genome as we have, they did better because their moderate lifestyle modified the way their genes expressed themselves in healthy outcomes. Despite the interventions of modern pharmacology and the elimination of animal fat and the swallowing of statin drugs, we have experienced increasingly bad health. The genes have not changed, but their effect on us has changed, and not for the good.

If you do not know what is wrong, you cannot fix it, and if nothing is wrong, you need to continuously improve it so that when the decline of age arrives, you have plenty in the storeroom, as our great grandparents and ancestors had. They might have died of infections, which are not a problem today, but they did not die as we now do, or suffer the same disabilities, the lifestyle-related big disabilities of today that are blowing out the medical budgets of most countries. And now, infectious diseases are fighting back and winning.

Measurement: if you are feeling a bit blue, is this worry, anxiety, or a mood problem? You just do not know, do you? How strong is your back, can you hold a crunch for three minutes, or a plank? What is a crunch, or a plank? You might not know. How variable is your heart rate beat-to-beat ratio? If yours is not great, you might have 500% the cardiac risk of another who does know and works on it. Is the bacterial content of your mouth raising the cardiac risk as we speak, as you chew on dried fruit, which you THINK is healthy? Is your backache a result of bone problems or of tightness of iliacus and psoas? You do not know. Is your sunblock helping you avoid melanoma, but causing Alzheimer's and osteoporosis? The creases in your earlobe and the pads of fat under your eyes, is that cardiac disease, or… not? That lack of knowledge will eventually kill you, after some prolonged misery.

So I have to ask you this question: how do you expect to age gracefully and be a healthy and strong eighty year old if you do not have a clue about how your brain or body is doing? And even if you run to your doctor, chances are he will not measure it either, as his focus will be on what he can treat, not what you have to manage on your own.

If you are in the United Kingdom and go to a doctor, or in the USA, or in India, or in Germany, going to a doctor to be assessed might elicit a completely different response. You might get a drug from one, a natural product from another, a chewing out from another about exercise, with or without any ideas about what to do, one might stick needles in your ear, and one might stick a needle in your butt. One might measure your *chakras*. Another teaches you *prana* breathing. It's all too confusing. Deprived of social support and real friends, you may fail to deal with natural grief, and be given an antidepressant that will not work in most people. And if it does work, it may be a placebo, not an active ingredient that does the trick. And if it does work, six months later it might stop working completely. Alternatively, you might go off it and within days decline into a horrible discontinuation syndrome. Aaargh!

So who is the expert in you and your life? And where do you find this person? Actually, you can find them anytime in the mirror.

The answer is that You are the expert in YOU. But you have to measure where you are at, NOW, at this stage of your life. You need to experience the magic of numbers.

You are the expert in You:

When it comes to a healthier lifestyle, you alone know how you have succeeded in the past and how you have failed. If you have tried to get healthier, stop biting your nails, or smoking, or get to the gym, or lose weight, or be nicer to your friends, you will know this kind of change can take a long time, can take several attempts, and you often waste time taking the wrong advice from the wrong person – or magazine. Or Doctor. Or guru. How did you know what was good advice, and how did you take it when you heard it? Or not?

If I do nothing else in this book, I hope at least to convince you that when it comes to changing your lifestyle for the better, No One, but NO ONE is coming to save you from yourself and your fate: when it comes to healthy change – you are IT. And that is not a bad thing. You are not alone in meeting healthy challenges when you have someone right next to you who knows you just as well as you know yourself, because it's you anyway.

> *One of the great drivers to a better life is the desire to guide your own existence, to keep control of your journey through life.*

This is the principal of *autonomy*. Even parents can get it wrong if they miss that about their children. At nineteen years old I approached my mother about my becoming a psychologist. The response kind of sunk me, and she was right in her reasoning. Later on in life, I did study to become a psychologist, and did okay, and I cannot think of having lived my life any other way. The advice my mother gave was correct, but that did not put me off forever. However, it did cause me to waste years of my time: the drive to guide our own destiny, to chart our course, to be in control of our day to day existence, is the strongest engine we have to motivate us, to guide our choices and to achieve happiness on our own terms, on our own merits. The 'self-made' person is always highly valued compared to someone who inherited it.

> *So this is why, when a doctor or guru or dietician gives us the best advice in the world, we just do not take it. We heed their advice, but their argument is never as potent as the one we might make to carry out something that really resonates with us. Making your own argument to change does work better than following someone else's advice.*

The problem with other people telling us what to do is that we are *living* our lives, somewhat alone, while they, including our mothers, are just *visiting* our lives for a short time, seeing only a cross-section, a snapshot of our lives – a moment in time. We know ourselves well, we are just often unable to watch our own lives happening, and measure and manage the fallout when we go wrong.

When you measure where you are now, from a body and brain perspective, you create a baseline against which you can measure how well you are charting a personal course towards feeling amazing each day. As my friend Mimma Mason says, personalized health begins with taking a baseline and managing the bits you need to. This baseline is the launch pad for taking charge of your own health.

I am not negating modern medicine. Measuring your colon with a colonoscopy is lifesaving, but avoiding bowel cancer has nothing to do with the doctor. Measuring your cholesterol may be a good idea, but treating it with a statin drug might not be the best way to avoid a heart attack. Being healthy but stressed or riddled with worry on a daily basis might kill you faster than fat in your blood, or your sugar intake. On the other hand, we were advised to avoid animal fats in our food, but that did not reduce the heart-disease risk over the past few decades, even though we listened, substituting margarine for butter, taking statins and so on. Emerging discussion on Paleo diets and the value or otherwise of taking statins or eating low fat, modified products is beginning to challenge the entire idea of avoiding natural food in favour of processed, reduced-fat foods, which may have increased our risk of obesity and heart disease, not reduced it.

We all know of peak athletes who have dropped dead during a marathon or on the soccer pitch: we ask ourselves how a 'perfectly healthy' young man could die like that? Well, the answer is that they were not 'perfectly healthy' and that measuring them simply as medicine routinely does might not cover all risks such as the stress of managing their huge incomes or competing in a vicious world or having poor heart rate variability.

Reading this book, you will cover six areas of life which you can measure and target for yourself, guiding yourself along each pathway to ensure you have the best life, which will ensure the perfect way of modifying your bad genes and enhancing your good ones, as far as is humanly possible. **You will learn how to become the expert in you**, measuring and managing all six areas to optimise body and brain.

Most experts you may consult with will have studied narrowly, focusing on what is critical only to their field. In this way, a cardiologist may encourage you to have a few alcoholic drinks a night. The dietician may scold you for the empty carbohydrates consumed, yet offer pickled cucumbers as 'free food' ignoring the salt content. A gastroenterologist might scold you for your attack on your liver and stomach lining, a neurologist on the damage done by enhancing GABA, which the brain responds to by activating Glutamate toxicity and your physician might direct you to red wine and dark chocolate. Your French friend seems to eat the richest food and stays thin as a rake, your Italian chef friend seems to live like a gourmet lunatic, but is chasing women at ninety-five. Your fit and healthy buddy drops dead on holiday by the sea at forty despite jogging twenty kilometres each day.

This means you have to look at everything, from the entire health prism, to keep the best things going and negate the bad. It might seem overwhelming but...

Little things make a big difference

An integrated approach takes the best out of all these worlds and asks you to filter the small things that make a big difference to your lifestyle. This does not mean finding another two hours a day to go to the health club, or go on a diet on and off, losing and gaining weight or eating unhealthy but 'free' foods. There are no stomach crunches, not a bench press in sight. Just good advice you CAN take.

Little things can make a big difference. In each of these six areas of body and brain optimisation, you will find ways to measure and manage these divisions of lifestyle, building resilience to the damage done by a modern lifestyle, to enhance bodies designed for an ancient world and for the brain that guides you each day.

There is a big difference between what you intend to do on 1 January, and what you actually do from 2 January onward. There is a huge difference between what people intend to do, and what they do eventually manage to do.

When you become an expert in You, you will know what to do, what little changes to adopt, which will have the best outcomes for you. This means real, meaningful, permanent changes without becoming a monk or eating like a rabbit, or 'shredding' your body at a gym, heaven forbid what that might mean, and certainly you may not be twenty years old and find that idea appealing.

This may be because you have not adopted to change freely or rather you try to comply with someone else's orders or requests, a doctor, a friend, a partner. This is all good advice that you just do not take. They are visiting your life, not living it, no matter how well-meaning.

Adopting small meaningful changes, which do make a difference, is a very different recipe for success compared to trying to comply with the orders of a dietician or doctor, or keep up with a friend. Compliance is not adoption and is often short lived.

Measuring where you are at and making a compelling argument for the small things you can do to change your health prospects in a big way is the key to success in building resilience to ageing in a modern world and in becoming the peak version of yourself. It is the key to success of kick-starting yourself in the right direction, not leaving it until some future Monday.

How and what do I measure?

One of the best overall measures for your vitality is to make a comparison between your chronological age and your biological age. Taking into account how big your waistline is, your cholesterol, your weight, your stress, food intake, sleep and other parameters adds up to a good estimate as to how you are doing risk-wise. Counting how many hours you sit for a day is vital.

My colleague Paul Taylor has developed a BioAge measure, which can be used to estimate your biological age and risk (see www.bioagetest.com). Say for instance you are forty years old, but your parameters as measured are a little worse than they should be; you might have a BioAge of forty-five and need to recover at least five years of your life from the dustbin.

Many of you have access to a Wellness or Vitality program at work, or via your health insurer, most of which have an online Health Risk Assessment, which is a good place to start entering your health data to see how you are doing.

The Mayo Clinic has one, Embody Health (**Google: Mayo Clinic Embody Health Portal**) and most medical insurance companies in the world also offer these.

For some strange reason, if data presented at DMEC conferences is anything to go on, only 10% of workers bother to use these facilities (see www.dmec.org). Even if incentivised by the boss to the tune of $100 Amex gift cards, most staff simply do not go in and use these valuable, expensively developed toolkits: why not? We will talk about that later.

Big health insurers in the USA have informative sites with all kinds of metric instruments, for all kinds of body measures, for instance, the My Optum Health site, which is part of United Health Group, is a personalized portal for clients with a huge library of stuff (**Google: My Optum Health Tools and Tips**).

Some companies bring it all together, to reward you for measuring and managing your lifestyle in large groups, a kind of wellness exchange, so have a look at Life Ally (**http://lifeally.com**) for a great example.

You get the idea. Measure, it, then manage it using the optimising approaches below as a guide.

So let us get going. I am going to start with the big one (groan). No, I am not talking about exercise… I mean movement. Movement in all three dimensions, movement to engage and foster body and brain connectedness. Evolving, novel movement, like a dancer learning new steps, keeping the brain engaged and watching, monitoring where the feet, hands, hips, ankles and buttocks are going, keeping things on an even keel, like constantly getting the conductor to pay attention to each and every artist in the orchestra. Movement, as I noted before, and thought share a common substrate, the motor cortices, and hence, the more novel your language of movement that evolves, the more your brain has to work smarter, just as if you were learning French or some other language for the first time. Such challenges recruit and stabilize new brain tissue, and foster resilience, vitality, and hope.

Chapter Two

orange

movement: it does not have to be an electric chair that executes you

ictor worked hard during the week; either in his office, on his computer, or in his car, driving to see clients to service their software. He made a fairly good living. Every night he set out on his jog, bashing the roads of his suburb and working up a good sweat to counter his stressful day. Setting off one night, past the beach, he felt a bit dizzy, only coming to his senses in a hospital four days later. At thirty-seven, he experienced sudden cardiac death, rescued by lifesavers coming off duty from the beach, luckily with access to a defibrillator. Loss of cardiac rhythm nearly killed him off.

Chances are, as you read this, you are doing the most deadly thing you can do, and which almost killed Victor off. It is increasingly a major health risk and by doing it, you are heralding a cascade of metabolic events linked to nearly every avoidable health complication known to modern science.

When you do it, your brain switches of, you start to burn only one calorie per minute, your lipase inhibitors, which protect you from dangerous fats drop to 10% of their capacity; electrical activity in the legs switches off, HDL 'cholesterol', which protects you, drops off, the risk of diabetes increases as insulin sensitivity drops off. Your cells become inflamed, leading to illness, including depression and brain decay. If you do this a lot, you begin to double your risk of heart disease and increase your chances of dying dramatically compared to someone who does not.

This awful activity? The worst thing you can do? It is known as **'Sitting Down'**.

If there is one thing you must change in your life, it is this single activity. We are just not engineered for sitting. The average adult spends 90% of their leisure time sitting, not just the time they spend at work. It does not mean that exercise is going to be able to reverse this, it means you seriously have to limit the time you spend sitting.

You might not want to take my word for it, so just look at some studies done recently. A current study in the *Archives of Internal Medicine* by Dr Hidde van der Ploeg and her colleagues found that adults who sit for about eleven hours a day, about as much as the average worker, have a 40% greater chance of dying than someone who does a lot less sitting. This was a study of 220 000 people in Australia: 5000 died in three years of the study, with at least 7% attributable to just sitting. Eight to eleven hours of sitting increased death risk by 15%. Is this new information? No: Ramazzini made this link between sitting and ill health in the 17th century. The British have known for the last fifty years that bus drivers die younger than postmen do.

A Finnish study, quoted by the Ratey Institute in March 2012, led by Finni and colleagues and published in the *Scandinavian Journal of Medicine and Science in Sports,* found that the muscles of workers who sit during the day are inactive for about 70% of their time, even if they do exercise. We were designed to use our muscles and move around most of the day, so this is just not a good scenario for body and brain as well. Designed for movement, we spend only 30% of our time moving around. Not good is it?

Women are at particular risk. A study in the *American Journal of Epidemiology* in 2010 by Patel and colleagues of over 123 000 people found that women who sat for more than six hours per day were 37% more likely to die than women who sat for less than three. That was the good news for women who were active. The BAD news is that for those women who sat more and were less active, that death risk increased to 94%. Sitting less and being more active was a lot less risky: even so, sitting overall increased the risk dramatically. By **Sitting, you are starting the process of dying!**

So the men reading this are feeling happy, right, it is only a risk for the women? Sorry boys: Tatiana Warren and her colleagues in the USA published their 2010 research on 7744 men from their twenties into their eighties. They measured the cardiovascular disease risk in men who rode in a car for more than ten hours a week, or sat doing various activities for more than twenty-three hours a week. Compared to guys who sat in cars for less than four hours a week, or less than eleven hours a week sitting doing all kinds of stuff, the death risk for the drivers was 82% worse and for general lazy bones was still 64% worse with everything else controlled for.

Sitting is fatal, eventually. Are you feeling happy that we take our kids, and after seven years of moving a lot, we plonk them down in chairs and tell them to shut up and NOT move for eight hours a day? And then send them home to not move and do their homework for two to four hours more? Okay, well they might not be doing their homework; however they just sit at their laptops and smart phones for eight hours more! And they sit for the next twelve years at school and another three to five at university, and then for seven to ten a day at work after that for the rest of their working lives? The way we do these things is surely madness.

This is killing them. Social Networking used to have a different name; it was called 'outside', where there was sun, and Vitamin D. Now there is nothing. By the time the average American kid reaches twenty-one, they will have spent 10 000 hours sitting and playing computer games, as much time as they spent in primary and middle school, so double the time sitting instead of playing outside and in doing so, changing their genomic expression for the worse.

Our genome evolved to move, so the first brain and body optimiser you need to consider is **movement**. Being sedentary for whatever reason is a killer in its own right, and it is not just cardiovascular disease you have to worry about. The inflammatory side to sitting and the downstream effects on the chemistry of the body have high-risk implications for Alzheimer's and everything else body and brain health related, including depressive illness.

The good news is that although movement will not change the underlying genetic structure of your body, it will change the way the genes express themselves, the effect they have, in the muscles that get moved enough. You can have a look at Barres and colleagues in the journal *Cell Metabolism* in March 7th 2012 working out of the prestigious Karolinska Institute, and see what movement can do for you, if applied frequently to break up your sitting time.

By the way, caffeine consumption can mimic the muscle contractions of movement, and I mention that again in the 'feed yourself' section.

So that is a win, but the muffin eaten with coffee might not be.

Steve Aldana is a professor of lifestyle medicine at Brigham Young University in Utah. He notes that 78% of workers are sedentary, and that 15% of the medical costs of a nation are caused by this lack of movement. Add in obesity and its effect on health and 35–40% of healthcare costs relate to lack of movement. If you do nothing else, movement is the biggest change you can focus on to achieve vitality, and save the nation's chequebook.

As you will see from my story about Victor above, I use the word 'movement' and I do not use the word 'exercise'. Victor exercised and was otherwise fit and healthy, but died suddenly and had to be resuscitated because of the problems related to his hours in the stressful car environment and in front of a computer, adding up to seventy hours a week. Lack of movement and recovery time, not lack of exercise *per se* killed him. The issue is how much we move in a day, not just how much is robust exercise. I will come back to that.

A 2012 study in the Journal, *Alzheimer's Disease*, based on research coming out of the University of South Florida and Fudan University, studying the elderly in Shanghai, found that the usual decline in brain volume, a risk for dementia, was not present in people practicing non-aerobic Tai Chi: brain volume in fact grew on MRI scan, and on neuropsychological tests, memory actually improved, as well as gains in other neuropsychological function. Ageing brain is thus not necessarily normal and irreversible, and certainly movement here, not aerobics, plays its part in keeping the body and brain essentially unchanged and even growing. This was only a small study of just 120 people, but imagine what a huge study of millions of Chinese might show?

The take-home message here is that not using the muscles of the arms, torso and legs for most of the day and night is likely to be more harmful than anything else you can do to yourself.

Sitting is the body's way of telling the brain it is time to start dying.

And we do not only sit at work or after retirement:

After a busy day in front of a telephone or computer or similar machinery or technology, most of us sit all the way home in a car or train, walk up the one step at the front of our house and collapse into a chair. We then get roused by the family cook to sit and consume a huge meal sitting at a table, and flop back into a chair to watch TV, stopping only to flop into bed. Should we go to a gym or health club, most of us will sit on some machine pushing levered weights around, or trample on a treadmill and get a bit of a sweat. Worse, we have all watched people circling the parking lot at the local health club looking for a place to park, so they can go and walk miles on the treadmill.

Oh, and by the way, that treadmill is NOT the same as walking on the road. Failure to push off with your back foot as you walk on a treadmill, which does not require glute-controlled push-off on each step, is going to ruin your butt muscles and hurt your lower back and ignore a lot of important brain activity that is not happening on a treadmill. Sitting in a standard, triple-flexed position the whole day tightens and stretches in the wrong place, and a treadmill will not fix that. Moving in just two dimensions can also be improved on. Think movement in a bubble in which you are centred: fill that bubble with movement, as you would with dance or Tai Chi.

While sitting with ankles, knees, hips and upper body triple-flexed, namely bent at an angle, muscles in the front of the pelvis tighten, the stomach tightens, the biggest muscle in the body, the diaphragm is compromised and it just is not a healthy position. The body and brain deteriorate.

So how is it that we get so 'tired' after sitting on our butts at work? We think it is the stress, the concentration, the focus of our busy day? Only partly, as essentially we are doing something we were never designed to do. Sitting is not using the entire brain body system to do what it was supposed to do, namely to work hard physically. Putting an elite fit athlete into a chair for ten days will just about ruin their muscle tone. Ordinary people will not do any better.

Without movement, the brain will not work well either. Mostly, the reason we arrive home after doing nothing physically exhausting but still feel so tired is a result of the lack of doing something physically exhilarating. And lack of movement is a feature of mental illness too. Lack of movement is connected to the rise of inflammation at the cellular level, and areas of the brain, confronted with lack of movement, excess sugar and Omega-6 oils are particular target areas for this inflammation.

Movement and the brain

With the chances of living a long life ahead of you and me, we have to make sure that we not only live a long time, but live long and healthily enough to enjoy life, and not spend it in a doctor's room or a hospital ward, a wheelchair, or a nursing home for dementing seniors. Refer to the study of the Shanghai Chinese I mention above, with their increased brain volume because of Tai Chi movement and other aspects of their lifestyle. This is impressive. Ageing has a slow-it-down solution: movement. And, more importantly, Tai Chi is movement in all three dimensions. Many of these people may not sit on chairs, but prefer to squat, which is also considered healthier (**Google: 'Asian Squat'**).

> *If there is a magic pill to take to avoid disability as you age, and I mean as you age past thirty or forty, you should take it, and there is: it is complex movement.*

Look at the teaching nun studies I mention elsewhere. These women are on the move constantly, apart from other things they do across the body brain spectrum to improve their lives using lifestyle elements that can be controlled.

John Ratey is a professor of psychiatry at Harvard Medical School no less. He wrote a very well quoted book entitled *Spark* in 2008 (you can follow him on Facebook via *'The Ratey Institute'*). The book was a major departure for Ratey from his previous works on personality disorder and other standard psychiatric stuff. Ratey in particular focused on the effects of exercise on the brain, and the resulting increase in brain growth factors and higher scores in standard tests for university entrance in the USA and other improved parameters. Really bad schools upped their nationwide profile simply by adding exercise to their school's curriculum.

What Ratey and others began to see in the scientific literature was that several growth hormones for the brain, those that help build brain tissue and those that help build the blood supply and nutrition for brain growth, and regulate blood sugar, are liberated by using the muscles in the body.

This means that movement is an effective strategy for keeping your body healthy, I am sure that you get that fact, but it ALSO and in some cases, more importantly, not only saves your body from movement: it does not have to be an electric chair that executes you

unhealthy decline, but also keeps your thinking and reasoning and other cognitive issues going at the right pace in your brain. To achieve this you have to sit less, and disrupt sitting patterns often for brain health as much as body integrity.

Arthur Kramer and colleagues in the influential journal *Nature* wrote in 1999 that training people to move robustly, such as aerobic exercise, improved how they used the major systems in the brain, the executive functions. These are the functions that support planning, making choices, solving problems, thinking, binding events across time, organizing and socializing and on and on to ensure success in what we plan to do. Compared to those who do not move like that, the aerobic group did so much better.

Carl Cotman and colleagues at the University of California showed that movement caused cascades of those growth factors I mentioned before. It also helped prevent the cellular inflammation that is part and parcel of cognitive decline and neurodegeneration: by this, we mean the dementias. Charles Hillman and colleagues went on to find the same in 2002, published in the journal *Psychophysiology*. And of course there are countless others who have found the same, as Ratey has spoken about.

The inflammation segment of this decline is caused, mostly, by a sedentary work and leisure lifestyle. This is not just cognitive decline as in dementia, but also in depression and other mental illnesses. Andrew Miller and colleagues, in the journal *Biological Psychiatry* reviewed this extensively in 2009. In *The New York Annals of the Academy of Science* in 2007, Bonita Marks and her colleagues wrote about the effect of such exercise on the integrity of the white matter of the brain, and using an Alzheimer's disease assessment tool, they found a twenty-six point improvement in the exercise group versus a decline of one point in those who did not move as much.

The rot starts early, decades before symptoms appear, and that is too late to do much to avert disaster. Early people, early!

So now you might be telling me you hate aerobic exercise. Well, for you, there is still hope. Hope comes in the form of a kind of movement called 'Interval Training'. For example, you might not be a runner (I confess, I am not). This means that if you are like me, you will need a 'quick fix'. The good news is that there is such a thing, in interval training. You can run flat out in a sprint until you run out of breath (for me, about 50-100 yards, or seven seconds of rapid foot movement on the spot at home). Then you stop running and walk slowly until you can breathe nicely again, and your heartbeat is back to normal. Then sprint flat out again, repeat the recovery time. Do this for fifteen minutes in the park or your yard, and you will have accomplished a lot. A 2009 article in the journal from *The American College of Cardiology* by Tyldum and colleagues found that interval training was even superior to aerobic exercise. So this high level effort versus recovery strategy saves you time, is easy to do, even if you just walk fast enough to achieve breathlessness and then recover, and probably has the same outcome as more sustained jogging or aerobic exercise, certainly from a cardiac point of view, and what is good for the heart is good for the brain too. You can see a recent review of this literature here: **Google: Physiological adaptations to low-volume, high-intensity interval training in health and disease.**

Movement is king when it comes to building resilience and a new you in the time available in a busy life, with low or high intensity interval training.

Rod Dishman and his colleagues, in the journal *Obesity* in 2006 concluded that training motor skills by regular movement enhanced executive functions of cognition and some types of learning, including motor learning in the spinal cord. They concluded that the adaptations in the central nervous system they observed have implications for the prevention and treatment of obesity, cancer, depression, the decline in cognition associated with aging, and neurological disorders such as Parkinson's disease, Alzheimer's dementia, ischemic stroke, and head and spinal cord injury. Regular movement means movement multiple times per day, disrupting your sitting time. See some more points on this below.

I hope I have made my point. Sitting leads to a decline in brain and in the functions of brain such as thinking and problem solving, and in the all too common realm of mental illnesses such as depression, as well as the more predictable and understandable effects on the body. Go figure – body and brain are one and the same, right?

Victor came in to see me for the first time, shattered. He just did not get it, what am I doing wrong? He never saw his weekly seventy hours of sitting as a risk factor, which wasn't attenuated by his jogging and overall fitness. When his bloods were done in hospital, his inflammatory markers were high, his cholesterol high, his blood pressure high, his scores on psychological and neuropsychological tests were even worse. He thought he was just stressed, which he was. The IT business had declined with the global financial collapse; he lost half his clients, the big ones. He was told to go home and rest after the hospital. He could not, and was restless and paced the floor. His wife said he was driving her nuts and was biting his nails, something she had never seen him do. His doctor diagnosed him with an anxiety and a mood disorder, and gave him medication, which helped him after three weeks, but stopped working after three months. He stopped the medication and three days later suffered a discontinuation syndrome, a type of withdrawal. He had to start taking the pills again, which ruined his sex drive, already depleted *by his mood and physical weakness, and sedated him all day. Unable to relax, forced to pace the floor, a side effect of the medication called akathisia, he decided to kill himself with his antidepressants, which just made him vomit. Then, on his birthday, his wife gave him a six month voucher for the local health club. "They saved my life".*

What kind of movement?

By now, you will be shouting at me, saying all very well and fine Dr Sugarman, but I have to sit for my job; I have to travel long distance in traffic just to get to work; I have to… blah blah… I understand that. There is a solution though. Remember, I am not in the business of trying to change your lifestyle in major ways, I know it is unlikely that you can do that, however:

There is now compelling evidence that just moving regularly, which breaks up your sedentary time, has great benefits. Healy and her colleagues, writing in the journal *Diabetes Care* in 2008, found those benefits. It is the act of prolonged sitting that is to blame, and that is something that you can change. It is not only about exercise as van der Ploeg and his colleagues have found, but by sitting less and for shorter periods of it. Yes, you have to exercise, but that is not enough, you have to move more and sit less as well: this is not negotiable, apparently. Do not let the dangerous act of sitting carry on uninterrupted.

Apart from regular, hourly movement, the interval training I mentioned above is also highly rated as a way to stay healthy enough to enjoy life through the lifespan. This means energizing yourself through movement to achieve more in the day at work and still go home with extra energy than before for the more important social interactions you will have at home with partner and kids. And your dog will love you when you take him to the park for some interval training. Alternatively, running full tilt on the spot, with hands pumping up and down in seven to ten second bursts is also effective.

Professor Maureen McDonald at McMaster University in Ontario has been investigating the effects of a high-intensity workout lasting thirty seconds at 100% of your recommended maximum heart rate, or sixty seconds at 90% (subtract your age from 220, and that is approximately your maximum heart rate: for a fifty-year-old, 170 or so). After the first minute, you relax for a minute again, and then do another one minute frenzied workout, and then relax, and do this until ten minutes of exercise and ten minutes recovery has passed. They concluded in their studies so far that this is as worthwhile as you can get. It appears that cardiac patients can manage this safely too as the input is so brief, and recovery good, that there is no risk demonstrated so far in their studies. You can, as I mentioned above, see references to this work elsewhere recently: **Google: Physiological adaptations to low-volume, high-intensity interval training in health and disease.**

Speak to your doctor though about doing this kind of exercise!

Incidental Movement

What saved Great Grandma from this bad sedentary stuff was largely incidental rather than planned movement. Pictures of my great grandparents seem to provide ample shapely evidence that they did not spend any time at the health club, and anyway there was no such thing for them. However, they did a lot of movement in their daily lives as I recall. They lived in small villages, they walked everywhere, and they worked behind counters in their shops: they rolled cigars, chopped up stuff, loaded and unloaded trucks and shelves, and ran away from Cossacks and so on. They moved all the time. Incidental movement is movement you do not plan, but is made a vital part of the daily life you lead. This is the opposite of planned movement, such as going to the gym. Incidental movement:

- It can mean commuting to work by train while standing, absorbing the pitch and yaw (that's rocking and rolling) of the train or ferry by flexing the leg muscles.

- It can mean cycling at least part of the way to work, or walking to work if you are so inclined.

- It can mean using the stairs everywhere, not the elevators.

- Using a wireless network printer on the other floor or other side of the office to yours, or the toilet two flights of stairs away from your usual one.

- It can mean installing a vibrating PowerPlate next to the water fountain.

- It can mean washing clothes by hand, hanging them up outside on the clothesline and washing them again each time it rains on them.

- It can mean cooking from scratch, standing in the kitchen, or watching TV while standing and ironing clothes.

- It can mean pacing the floor using a headset for phone calls.

- It can mean purchasing a standing desk for home or work.

- It can mean spending hours dancing to nice music with your partner, instead of watching TV or a movie, which is how I spent my teenage years when people came to play.

- It can mean having no internet at home, no computer, and swopping the Blackberry for blueberries.

- Take the arms off your typing stool, so that each time you get up you only use your legs.

- It can mean finding a tree at the park, and chasing your dog around it, playing this way and that.

- It can mean just seven seconds of high-speed running on the spot lifting the legs high and stepping as softly and in the most controlled manner you can.

- It can mean walking to, and using, the local convenience store and carrying the parcels home each day, instead of driving to the mall once a week. Helps you cook from scratch each day too.

- It can mean anything. Any movement you have built in to your day. Every little bit counts.

Most importantly, when your daily work or home life involves prolonged sitting, avoid doing it continuously for more than fifty-five minutes or so. Stand up and move at least that often.

Here are a few movements you can try to overcome the nasty, dangerous, debilitating effects of sitting:

1. Stand up, one foot forward, one behind, about three-foot lengths apart. Let your body sag straight down, keeping it vertical, hands loose at the side. Do not lunge too deep, keep it slow and steady. Rhythmically rise up and drop down until the back knee gets close to the ground. Support yourself with one hand on the desk if you need

to help balance. Do this for five counts with each leg forward, so ten in all. Increase this by one count per day until you are doing about twenty or so. Keep it slow, and limit the range to keep it comfortable. Do this at least once an hour.

2. Stand up straight, arms by the side. Take a short step forward and at the same time, raise both arms into a vertical stretch, turning the thumbs of the outstretched hands inward, so the palms face each other. As you move forward, and as the arms come straight up, let the knees bend slightly so the body drops just a little. Step back upright again, arms by your sides. Move slowly and limit the range of movement, repeating these five times for each leg to start, increasing by one a day until twenty each side are accomplished. Keep the body straight, the back long.

3. Stand up straight, legs at shoulder width. Raise right arm up. Now reach over and down to the left, while moving the right foot to a T position across the toe of the left, touching down as far behind the left foot as possible. Come up and past the original upright position stepping around until the right foot is at 90% to the original position, stepping out to the right, the right hand raised high and back as far as possible. Repeat eight to ten times, then swop to the right-hand side and repeat.

4. Do number one above again, but this time lean forward at about thirty degrees to engage the gluteal muscles a bit more. I prefer the bolt upright position though, you choose.

5. Lean against the wall, hands at shoulder height. Feet parallel and 90deg to the wall. Raise one leg until the thigh is parallel to the floor, the leg hanging vertically. Swing the raised leg to left and right slowly, enjoying a full range of side to side movement, but don't push the limits. Let the shoulder blades work with the upper back and knees soft. Move the hips with the leg as it goes outward. Swap legs.

6. Move rapidly in any direction, even sideways, for seven seconds at a time. Think of being in a bubble and of filling it with movement of hands and feet, as you would in Tai Chi. Think of the kind of movement you would do to attract a helicopter in to the mountain where you are stranded, if you know what I mean!

7. Buy a balance board and stand on it while brushing your teeth and washing your face or the dishes.

Go on to YouTube and type in the search engine 'functional movement exercises' or 'mobilizers' and choose some which make sense to you. Consult a personal trainer, who can advise you. Do Tai Chi.

To quote the great Jack Lalanne (look him up on YouTube as well), get moving. Jack knew this in the early forties and went on to live to ninety-six, relying on movement as one of the most important guarantees of a health future. And yes, his final death did harm his reputation, as he expected! He may not have been immortal, but he lived his life to his dying day in peak condition.

Turning to my colleagues in the USA, you can go to **www.coreperformance.com** and join for free. There are a host of videos and other information about getting moving in a great way, and doing so in your own time, when you find the time. I suggest you find time hourly and spend just a few minutes each hour saving your life.

Start the day moving: hit the ground running

When you wake up in the morning, do not hit the snooze button: move. There is evidence that during the snooze period you put your brain into a nasty semi-sleep which does not easily lift, worsening your day. What you can do, and, which will guarantee a better start to the day for your brain and body instead of snoozing, is to do some complex movements such as those above to wake up your brain and reconnect it to your body. As you will find out later, your brain has been doing some heavy lifting all night long, and from the early hours of the morning, your levels of the stress hormone cortisol, extremely inflammatory on its own, have been steadily rising. Moving first thing in the day helps a lot.

Penn State researchers have found that motor activity has a great spinoff in terms of creating a feeling of excitement and enthusiasm for life, as published in a 2012 edition of *The Journal of Sport and Exercise Psychology* by Amanda Hyde and her colleagues. So beginning your day this way is a good way to get going and improve your motivation if you are not a morning person. Oh, and later, you will see that a morning piece of chocolate cake can help you smile, as well as lose weight: I promise: this is what Israeli diet researchers have found.

Now while on that subject, here is the thing about cortisol. It is a stress regulating hormone, and one of the things that raises it sky high is robust, hard, exercise. Exercise is a stress on your body, but it is highly desirable that you do heavy exercise (such as Victor did) and you have to do some damage to muscle during exercise to release the nice growth hormones. Essentially however, too much heavy work is likely to cause injury and inflammation at the cellular level that is not desirable. Recovery is the key.

> *When you finish a bout of robust exercise, your body is way, way, less healthy then it was when you started.*

During recovery is when the health building process ramps up. Cortisol builds up while you are sleeping, peaking at 3am or so, so move when you awaken!

Recovery

What you now read is crucial.

The exercise fanatics you know are often plagued by injury, which sets them back. Great sportsmen and women have had frequent interruptions and sometimes ended their careers because of injury. Overtraining is so bad for you that one episode of overtraining can set my athletes back six months in their peak performance. Doing hectic training, you may run the risk of depleting essential amino acids and so the body gets them from cartilage and bone, causing injury and damaging your immune system.

> *It is during the recovery period that follows that the brain and body do their building and compensation, super-compensating with muscle and brain growth, if left alone long enough.*

Training on the tired muscle or brain leads to worse performance, and as noted above, injury and even burnout.

Here is the news about brain: your brain is not a muscle, and does not store energy. To replenish itself, it must rest, and preferably do only light lifting until recovered. Worked and recovered in cycles, both brain and body grow. You have to recover as much as you work, the one helping the other grow your body and brain resilience. It is like interval training: push and relax.

Timing regeneration and recovery are part of what we do in elite coaching. It is not a philosophical issue, it is vital to peak performers so that they can build on and then exceed previous levels of performance. Have a look at what Michael Kellmann wrote on the subject on this site: **Google: Michael Kellman Under-recovery and Overtraining.**

Recovery means doing movement that is not as intense. For the runner, this means walking, for the body builder, this means stretching; for athletes, this means ice, heat, massage, rest, elevation, using a foam roller (the Pilates kind), a massage stick, trigger point release, Tai Chi, Qi Kung and so on. Regeneration nutrition is another issue. So think again of the Shanghai Chinese with their diet, Confucian mindset, family ties, and Tai Chi among other elements of their lifestyle, all part of recovery from the demands of daily life.

Measuring Movement to Manage it:

I mentioned earlier that we can measure this and other aspects of health. Here is how.

Draw up a table labelled Monday-Sunday. Keep this up for a week, and just before bedtime, add up all the hours you sat in:

1. A motor vehicle: it must be less than ten a week or one and a half hours a day

2. A desk at work and

3. A chair at home: these two should not exceed three hours and fifteen minutes a day

Big Goal to Strive for to Save your life: to spend less than four hours a day, or less than ten hours a week in a car, or less than twenty-three hours a week sitting in all places, work or home. Wear a pedometer, and think of the thousands of steps you take a day. An office worker might manage 1500, or at best 3000-3500 steps a day, tops. You need more than double that just to keep the clock ticking, and our ancestors clearly did 10 000 to 11 000 steps a day. Hunters in the

Kalahari are closer to 70-80 000 a day, as we were designed to do. So a pedometer should show you walking about six to seven kilometres a day, just under four to five miles a day. That is essential. Stairs, road walking, interval training, these are all good to add to the pedometer. An accelerometer might also help you measure the effort you put into those steps, but either way, a cheap investment in a movement detector, or the use of one on your smartphone, Adidas MiCoach, Nike+ and iPhone, all of which are really simple and effective ways to measure and monitor your movement health.

Small Goal You Might Manage: Stand up (or get out of car) every forty-five minutes and spend one to two minutes mobilizing, stretching, moving or standing on a vibration plate such as a PowerPlate, or a balancing disk or board. Stand up without using your hands on the arms of the chair. That might amount to seventy leg presses a day in just getting you up off the chair.

What about the REALLY elderly?

Recently, my colleagues and I were confronted with a series of elderly folk in wheelchairs, or largely sedentary in a retirement village. On our TV show, we gathered a bunch of them in a room and got them moving. For the elderly, you would not imagine push-ups are a great exercise. However, move your thinking out of the box that has grandma lying prone on the ground struggling to push. We move them to a wall, against which they stand and lean. Then they push away, then relax back to the wall, then push away. Supported by one hand on the wall, they reach up, reach down, reach across, do soft knee bends. The body loves this. Moving the feet further away from the wall as they gain strength will increase the loading on them.

What about those in a chair, or using a walker? My colleagues are working hard with such people, playing balloon tennis and tossing squash or tennis balls at them, creating easily managed 3-D incidental movement. The brain stimulation is great: how far would a really aged person have to walk to increase their brain connectedness dramatically, perhaps by up to 30%? Studies have shown that just 600 yards a day would do that brilliantly in a few months.

So when we age, there is a natural decline in our muscles, right? Wrong. Dr Vonda Wright, at the University of Pittsburgh Medical Centre made the point in 2011 that older athletes are as strong as the younger ones, with only slight reduction in strength after sixty, and with no difference between sixty year olds and seventy and eighty year olds. She says it is inactivity, not age that causes the decline we see in the elderly. Canadian researchers in 2010 had found that continuous movement kept muscles from declining well into the seventies. Dr Wright will tell you if you ask her that through movement you can preserve muscle mass and strength and avoid the decline from vitality to frailty.

Using our muscles not only builds up energy by increasing the mitochondria, the power houses of the cells in the muscles, but it has the same effect in our brains making them faster and more efficient, or so says Dr Mark Davis from the University of South Carolina, in a recent article in *The Journal of Applied Physiology*. He notes that the evidence is accumulating that exercise keeps not just the body young, but the brain younger as well.

And yet again, look at *The Journal of Alzheimer's Disease*, and see what keeps the ageing Shanghai brain not just alive, but growing and functionally intact: Tai Chi, 3D movement, movement in all planes. Easy to do, every day. Your excuse…? Seems less compelling a reason not to live longer with an intact body and brain, yes?

For those of you who do work out, in between your exercises you need to mobilize; make sure you are not just ramming cortisol into your system without recourse to downtime. Active Downtime is not lost time: recovery builds on the foundation you laid with hard exercise. When you follow hard exercise with soft movement, recovery, you reap the benefits, not otherwise.

If you forget to move it, you will lose it. It is in your hands; decline is not a result of ageing, not much anyway. You make the difference, or you do not. It is your choice to age badly, to sit, to decline as the years pass. Do not blame age; you are the expert here, so you choose how you will age. And remember, the rot starts early, as we shall see again later. Move it. As you will recall from once being a child, movement was all about fun, chasing, catching, wrestling, even as a teenager with your little crush, tickling and wrestling were good precursors to desire, to living life and loving it. It does not have to decline with age, but it does, if age means inactive, sick, despairing. UGH!

Chapter Three

ye__ow

if you are what you eat, then you, dear friend, are eating your last meals, every day!

Jack, at seventy-five, was sent by his dietician. His weight fluctuated from ninety kilograms down to eighty-two, but despite sticking to his diet, he could not get his weight down to the seventy-six kilograms that she had indicated was necessary to reduce his reliance on medication for his type II diabetes, statin drugs, blood pressure medication, and painkillers for his arthritis. An architect until he retired, he had spent little time on site, but hours at his drawing table, leaving it to others to do the hands on building work. He had retired at sixty-five, well off financially, but his health had continued to decline since then. He travelled extensively with his wife, until she died of heart failure related to diabetes when she was sixty-eight. When she died, he weighed one hundred and fifteen kilograms. I noted he snacked on popcorn, as suggested by the dietician. He drank diet colas as suggested by his dietician, ate low fat food and milk, low sugar muffins and jelly, and avoided high GI foods. He ate fruit as snacks, and had swopped fizzy soft drinks for fruit juice. He snacked on pickled cucumbers, also suggested by his dietician as 'free food' when he needed something spicy. He walked two miles a day with a friend, Marty, and he enjoyed their chats. He ate a lot of greens each day, and a lot of protein in the form of steak and lamb, grilled on his barbeque at home. He used multivitamin tablets and avoided carbohydrates. He had lost twenty-five kilograms, but still needed to lose more.

Modern food is incompatible with human life. Jack Lalanne noted in 1940 that if God made it, eat it, but if man made it, leave it alone. Because you can chew or gulp something down does not make it food or even edible. If food is medicine, then modern processed food is poison. Human interference in food manufacture renders it no longer food. Of the hundreds of thousands of products on supermarket food shelves, perhaps only one hundred are edible by these standards. The food in a garage store is likely to not even remotely represent food as it might be, but rather it is closer to being like plastic or slow poison.

If you stare a doughnut in the face, it cannot reveal that once, somewhere, it was alive, or grew. Stare a carrot in the face: it looks like it was once alive. It stopped being alive when we picked it, but we do not have it in our back yard, so we hope it was picked recently. Since it once lived and grew, it was in balance with nature, and so with us. Many vegetables are toxic, such as the cruciferous ones, but our bodies were designed to respond to the toxic challenge of vegetables with improved health. My cat, not so much. My dog will eat anything. If my cat ate what my dog eats, it would die, soon. Look at the coffee bean: it is now roasted and processed, but you can see what it was when alive, and so when you crush it and heat it up in water, it is delicious, contracts your muscles, revs up your brain. Decaf, not so much: too much human interference.

And so it is with us. Processed food, modern food, stuff we buy in packets and cook or eat as they come, stuff with shelf lives until 2096, this is not food. You would not feed your Maserati fuel tank with this garbage, so why do it to yourself?

Two problems: time and yumminess. We use processed food because we lack the time to cook from scratch, and we get our brain taste and reward centres hijacked by addictive stuff in food. Fresh food in the USA used to be grown near Eastern cities, but soon farmers were further west, so they resorted to growing transportable grains, which could travel, unseating fruit and vegetables which could not do so well over those distances. This changed us.

Nutrition then and Now: Paleo Diet?

From ancient humans to modern humans, there was a 300% increase in the size of the brain, and more exactly, in the outer areas of the brain, making us more human than earlier hominids. We gained more language and more reasoning and more ability to simulate the best outcomes for us, based on actions we took now. A great system, but subject to error. Subject to hijacking by substances we never consumed, or were in short supply.

Salt and sugar were not unknown, but hard to come by. Earning your salt, a phrase meaning being worth your money at work, derived from Romans – being paid in salt, which was an expensive commodity. The British Government in India forbade native Indians from making salt; they had to buy it from British traders, because it was so expensive and lucrative. Sugar had to be grown from sugarcane, and otherwise was unknown, and like high-fructose syrup made from corn, has a high profitability for the manufacturers. We pay the price for that financial return with our lives. This means healthier, less transportable and less lucrative crops suffer, leading to shortages, e.g. rice in the east, when we grow corn for ethanol for instance, not food. We can get fresh food across long distance in USA and Australia, but it increases the cost way beyond a Big Mac.

The earlier humans also of course did not eat grain fed cattle, nor did they focus on only the choice cuts: they ate the whole animal, including the organs or sweet meats. Ugh. Some doctors are now adding offal into their patient's diets, as a treatment for multiple sclerosis.

So what did we eat, centuries and even thousands of years ago? We hear a lot today about so-called Paleo diets, or primitive food, hunter-gatherer diets, which presume that we evolved in some way to eat an ancient diet of food we could scavenge. These theories must be at least partly correct, but the problem with that one is that largely the environment and circumstances dictated diet, not evolution. So people who lived by the sea ate fish and seafood primarily, those inland less so, apart from perhaps bartering for dried fish inland. But most fishermen were fishing for subsistence and without refrigerators, and were largely like Unhygienix of Asterix cartoon fame, a fishmonger with really *smelly* stock!

Those inland would eat carcasses and roots taken from the soil, and learned to cook them so they did not die from the toxins, so manioc, cassava, yams, became their food. Once they learned to grow and harvest grasses, then grains became part of that. This meant they could farm cows and goats and add dairy to their diets. We also clearly evolved in forests, where small animals, insects and other food were available. Adding milk products and grain products created adaptations which plague some people today, for instance with lactose intolerance, irritable bowel syndrome, diverticulitis and other issues.

If you want to see a particularly compelling argument on the Paleo Diet, watch this on TED.com and you tell me what you think about the value of eating way beyond the modern diet: **Google: Terry Wahls Youtube Video.**

Dr Terry Wahls, in this video, makes a compelling argument for feeding your mitochondria, the power packs that drive your cells at the micro level.

Another caveat in Paleo or other, one-size-fits-all diets, is the issue of genetics. While the heavy red meat, high fat diet may suit some, it may be unwise in some others. In Jews for instance, with a history of intermarriage while confined to some small areas in Ghettos across the centuries in Eastern Europe, some diseases such as bowel cancer occur with higher frequency, making a Paleo diet ill-advised at this time owing to the connections with red meat. Healthy, fit, active young people may push this diet, but what of us, the elderly?

People on small islands such as Okinawa habitually eat primitive diets as they have a background where they could grow vegetables, fertilized with faeces and urine, eat fish they could catch and seafood they could harvest, some of which might not suit Western tastes.

This is partly why the Okinawans have more people living past one hundred than any other group in the world. And they have less breast, ovarian, colon and prostate cancer. They still adhere to a traditional diet. What makes the Okinawans such an interesting group to work with is that many of their families emigrated to Hawaii and Brazil. Did this make a difference? Yes, big time. Those who went to Brazil can live up to seventeen years LESS. And those who moved to Hawaii may live even longer than their first degree relatives in Okinawa. Why you may ask? There is more salt in the Brazilian diet and less salt and less soy sauce in the Hawaiian diet. Of course, less physical exercise, less fibre, less Omega 3 fat and more trans-fatty acids and Omega 6, higher body fat, lower flavonoid intake (antioxidants in fresh food), and less human interference in their food from ground or sea to stomach. It is as simple as that. Paleo diets are high in animal fat, low in grains and carbs, high in vegetables, coconut oil, and so on. The presumption is that the effect on cholesterol or cardiac risk does not exist in those living an active physical life. More so, they consumed vast amounts of vegetables, let's say about three plates a day of green leaves, as well as food that contained sulphur, vitamins of all kinds, Co-enzyme Q10, selenium, and other nutrients essential to body and brain, and of course animal and plant oils and fat. Processed carbs came later.

Recently we examined a sportsman group for overall bodily health at a cellular level using Spectracell analysis. One single athlete was optimal, compared to the optimal levels for just an ordinary citizen, let alone a peak athlete. The stunning finding was that this young man was the only vegetarian in the group, and a vegan to boot! It was clearly not his diet that was to credit for this achievement as much as his attention to what he eats. Vegans have to be careful to balance their diet for nutrients and so his involvement in what he ate and how much he ate of each food group within his ambit made him incredibly healthy. This was especially so in regard to the dangers of inflammation at a cellular level, as mentioned in the previous chapter.

Cellular inflammation from a food source is a real danger, especially in processed food overwhelmed with refined sugar, salt and oils/fat such as Omega 6. While Omega 6 is healthy, and necessary, the quantity consumed is highly elevated in our modern dietary intake when compared to Omega 3, given the processing of food that then produces this in excess. These two so-called eicosanoids need to be in balance with each other, at about three Omega 6's to two Omega

3's, not the current 20:1 in the USA, or about 15:1 in Australia. There is no doubt that the fact these two countries are in the grip of obesity, diabetes, Alzheimer's, depression and other avoidable illness pandemics, is partly to be blamed on overconsumption of Omega 6, as well as the excess consumption of refined sugar products, and also salt to a lesser extent. Omega 3 is anti-inflammatory, as are aspirin and statin drugs, but Omega 6 is pro-inflammatory at the cellular level. Combined with a sedentary lifestyle, the outcomes are poor.

Overconsumption of sugar is a nightmare. Some authorities are calling for it to be regulated or banned in some settings, as is another form of sugar – alcohol. Sugar is increasingly implicated in just about everything that is wrong with us, in modern food terms. Not all sugar is considered dangerous. It's the Fructose that is under suspicion, not in itself dangerous, but in the amounts we now consume it, it may be. The issue here of course is that all food and alcohol is sugar in some form or other. Not the white sugar cubes you find in restaurants, but the kind you find in carbohydrate and other food. We run on sugar, called glycogen, which just happens to be the real energy we use to propel our bodies and feed our brains. It is easy to get the sugar out of carbs, hard to get out of protein, but that just makes protein a better bet for losing weight and increasing cortisol. It is not about the sugar. It is about how much refined sugars we consume and how much humans have interfered with it.

Is it not something else? Why are we getting fatter and less healthy?

Well, the genetics of human beings have not shifted in the last thirty years. During that time however, obesity among school-going children has tripled. Meat and animal fat consumption has decreased, but heart disease rates have not come down accordingly. Statin consumption is up with debatable outcomes.

Behavioural factors are thus the only real cause here: issues like serving size, both for food and beverages, eating meals away from home, frequent snacking on energy dense foods, and consuming liquids with too much refined sugar, with liquid food being less satisfying (chewing tells our brain something about the fact we are eating, which helps satisfy hunger), and finally, the content of what we think of as tasty food in terms of unhealthy, man-altered substances is lethal. Giving children such food as 'treats' is arguably child abuse.

As I mentioned before, being sedentary is a risk, but other aspects of sitting while eating are also problematic. We consume more food while silent and watching TV, less if we are talking to others without the TV on. Sitting with TV, computers or smart phones/games in our laps displaces time we could spend outside and moving. It lowers our metabolic rate so we consume less energy and have more snacks. Finally, we are influenced to less healthy eating by ads on TV, which of course are selling processed food. Sitting is also most commonly indoors, and so we spend less time outdoors, and when we do, we are sun-blocked and clothed to avoid the harsh modern sun. The result: less vital Vitamin D in all of us, especially in children and older adults, and a link to MS, Autism and other conditions.

Processed Water

It is not just food. Water has become a processed commodity too. We consume too little water, and much of what we are consuming today is out of plastic bottles. Apart from this danger, add the adverse effects of the huge amount of factory water and non-renewable petroleum used to make the bottles and the litter pollution this manufacture and disposal creates for the planet. The actual bottle itself is producing bisphenol-a, an apparently nasty chemical under investigation at this time, with the FDA in the USA about to deliver a decision within a week at the time of writing. It too has been implicated in obesity, believed to affect unborn foetuses, and now found in the urine of 93% of Americans over the age of six. This may also be the lining the tins of canned food in many cases.

The absence of fluoride in bottled water has produced an increase in dental caries in bottled water fanatics, which has another health risk: dental caries and heart disease are linked. So floss, see the dentist regularly, and ditch the bottled water for water from the tap, in a glass or glass bottle. Metal food or beverage cans also contain the bisphenol as well as some sports equipment.

People generally are mildly dehydrated, with most accepting urine as a dark yellow: clear or vaguely straw coloured would be healthier. So for a 100lb adult, the minimum required to keep the basic metabolism healthily hydrated would be 50oz a day, using half the body weight and changing the lbs. to oz.'s, or the equivalent of about 300ml for each ten kilogram of body weight. So a sixty kilogram man would need about 1.8lit of water a day, more if he were training hard. A woman might need more than that, say 350ml per ten kilograms of weight. As the Israeli radio jingle went: "Drink cool refreshing water, there's nothing better for you, they say, drink water toooodaaaaaaaayyyy" or something similar. Good advice anyway.

For those who work out fanatically, or run marathons, or do twenty kilometres a day, the opposite may be true as well, the risk of **over-hydration** is quite worrying. Tim Noakes, a much published Professor from the University of Cape Town has had much to say about hydration over the years, and the risk of hyponatremia, namely the washing out of sodium (as in salt) by consuming too much water. Few of us have that risk, but read what he has to say anyway: **Google: Tim Noakes on overhydration in athletes Health24.**

Eating until you are not entirely full.

The Okinawan people have another advantage, which gives them a longer, healthier life with less risk of cancers: *Hara Hachi Bu*. This is the concept of eating until only 80% of hunger has been assuaged, meaning you stop eating before you are full, while you are still a bit hungry, not entirely stuffed or satiated. A restricted calorie diet has been associated with a longer lifespan, certainly in animal models anyway, citing fibroblast growth factor-21 as a factor.

This food reduction is literally necessary from the cradle to the grave. Infant's food may be laced with sugars hidden in different guises, including high-fructose corn syrup and other cheap and nasty forms of energy. Breakfast cereals are also sometimes referred to as 'breakfast desserts' more than real food, needing supplementation with vitamins and iron because they are so poor in natural nutrition. The CO_2 increase in our planet may rob modern plants of many of their nutrient concentrations as scientists are showing in experiments in crop growing where they pump CO_2 into the air around growing plants.

Fat cellular insertion into our bodies occurs in crucial periods, so by the end of puberty you are pretty much saddled with the fat cells you have, and will keep. Only filling or emptying them is now possible. You are what you stuff your face with.

Diets

When I talk about what you eat killing you, I am not talking about diets, or being on a diet, I am talking about food as fuel and food as medicine, as an alternative to food as being a poison.

Diets do work, and I think overall most diets work, if the goal is to lose weight. Losing or gaining weight may be a result of genetic interactions with eating, but as I noted before, this weight issue may be an epigenetic effect of eating the wrong food, in incorrect quantities, most of it 'modern' and highly processed, with not just junk food fitting that description, and not just over consumption of calories with less movement.

The issue with diets, even if they work, is that they usually do not constitute a lifestyle, and are therefore not sustainable. All diets must end, and the result is often a yo-yo effect with increased weight gain.

Low food input can trigger more cortisol, the hormone of stress and famine, one of the few chronic stressors ancient man had to contend with. You can ignore carbs, but digesting protein alone for instance can increase cortisol levels. Your metabolism changes in response to the restricted diet, leading the body to become even more efficient and needing less food: Weight Watchers clients often refer to how much food they are required to eat, not less. The brain and body can be really thrifty if they have to. Eating less frequently leads to trouble, including mood slumps associated with low carbohydrate intake, and kidney and other problems in high protein diets in those who are vulnerable. In other circumstances, the body might not process carbohydrate well, and prefer high protein if the body is to avoid diabetes in some people, with little carbs and lots of oil and fat in the diet, as suggested by Prof Tim Noakes and others. Fat certainly is the first content in food to switch off the hunger switches in the brain; there is nothing like fat, not protein nor carbs, that satisfies our hunger as quickly. The Paleo Diet depends on that.

The human body is referred to as 'thrifty', meaning it requires very little food to survive, long after water deprivation would have killed the animal. A single yoghurt may take seemingly forever to eliminate on a treadmill or bicycle in the gym, so neither exercise nor diet is going to do much on its own. A more complex and integrated approach is necessary to achieve health and a sustainable weight, if that is the goal. One hundred minutes of jogging might be required to eliminate the caloric intake of a single burger.

So if you are thinking diet, you have to think short-term. Alternatively, eating only food that has not been tampered with by humans, or stored too long, or poisoned with insecticides is not a diet, it is a long term lifestyle likely to show benefits when combined with a healthy lifestyle overall. Not one silo, many siloes. That is the value of the science of integration.

So let's go back to Jack. Poor old Jack. Jack was making mistakes that you should now be able to work out for yourself:

- *Jack was eating a lot of protein. The body has to work hard on extracting glycogen from animal muscle as food, and so this is a good strategy for losing weight but a bad one for inflammatory cortisol, compared to the ready energy one can get from carbohydrate. Trouble is, Jack was spending good money on grain fed beef, and highly marbled, fatty beef at that, high in inflammatory Omega 6's as opposed to grass-fed beef or lamb, which tends to have a balance of 3's and 6's. Overall, he was using margarine and other processed foods rich in Omega 6's to the extent his ratio of Omega 6 to 3 was not 3:2, but rather 25:1. At a cellular level this was a major threat to him.*

- Jack was not hydrating much, and when he was, he relied on diet soda, coffee with milk and artificial sweetener and soft drinks in general. This input of intense sweetness was triggering his brain and pancreas to release high doses of insulin to cope with what the brain thought was sugar. It also reset his brain chemistry to respond differently to real sugar, as he became increasingly insulin resistant, placing him at risk for worsening diabetes and later dementia. There is nothing healthy about diet soft drinks or diet food in general.

- Jack was walking with his friend, chatting away: this meant he was not becoming breathless. His workout of walking was burning some calories, but not much else, and certainly he was not doing any good to his overall muscle and brain systems compared to someone doing interval training or sweating up a storm at the gym.

- Jack was relying on highly processed vegetables, using oven chips as a source of potatoes, and eating high levels of refined fat in the oven chips and in microwave popcorn (30% fat) as opposed to cooking a healthy chip, or home oil – or air – popped corn. High levels of sodium and acid in the pickled cucumbers did not help either. Focusing on weight loss was not doing him any good. Cooking with olive oil was also an issue, as the olive oil was breaking down at low temperatures, becoming rancid. He would have done better with canola or avocado oil.

- His vegetable consumption came from supermarket food and most of it highly contentious as to when it was picked or shipped. He was sticking to juicing his raw vegetable and fruit, and tossing the fibre, which came out the other end of the juicer. His consumption of fruit juice exceeded the two fruit portions a day he should have consumed, perhaps up to ten fruits a day: without fibre, juiced fruit is just high volumes of sugar with good public relations appeal.

- Jack was eating low fat muffins: this translates as high sugar muffins. When he swapped to low sugar muffins, he unwittingly consumed two patties of butter for each muffin. Neither of these is good for him in the quantities consumed, increasing his weight or maintaining it. One muffin undid all his walking calorie gain.

- Jack was eating low glycaemic index foods unwisely. Low GI does not mean much for instance in his smearing his bread with low GI hazel nut paste: this is high in fat. The glycaemic index of watermelon is high, for instance, but the glycaemic load, the amount of glucose it delivers per serving is low. His teaspoon of chocolaty hazel nut paste is equivalent in terms of sugar delivered to TWO whole watermelons.

- Jack knew coffee was often better than tea as an antioxidant. However, his cappuccinos each day, loaded with milk and some sugar or sweetener raised his calorie count, as did his treat of a chocolate biscuit a day. Cutting these down was worth five kg in one year.

- Jack supplemented his regime with antioxidants in pill form. This is useless and a waste of money, as well as adding calories. In a vitamin tablet there might be forty ingredients; in a piece of healthy fruit or vegetables, there could be 30-40,000 nutrients. Antioxidants can be deadly in overdose, pill format.

- Jack's avoidance of carbohydrates entirely in the face of a metabolism which struggled to extract nutrition from protein, and his weak kidney function, led to him being placed on antidepressants, and constantly being out of energy, constipated, and his breath smelled. His cortisol and noradrenaline levels rose.

- Jack ate alone, and in front of the TV, or while using his iPhone or iPad. This led to his over consumption of calories, rather than a mindful approach to eating.

- Jack snacked on dried fruit: it was pointed out to him that the intense sugar content was ruining his teeth; as he chewed on it, the bacterial count in his mouth grew exponentially and this carried another cardiac risk, apart from weight gain. He also had bladder problems, which resulted in his consumption of dried cranberries: a small bag a day added 500 calories to his diet without him noticing.

- Jack's favourite breakfast cereal contained five whole grains. This was nice, except only 74% of the cereal was wholegrain if you read the box. The rest was sugar and salt, and most of it was dried fruit. Adding his cranberries, and the pecans he ate for his prostate issues, were a lot of calories.

The problem with refined sugar: Fructose is a culprit it seems?

"Sugar is a type of bodily fuel, yes, but your body runs about as well on it as a car would" – V.L. Allineare

Recently, together with most of the US Soccer National Men's Team and their coaches, I stuffed my face with cheesecake. This cheesecake, provided by Dr Kurt Mosetter from Zurich, was saturated with 'sugar', namely galactose, ribose, isomaltulose, erythritol, as well as almond and coconut flour, lactose free cream and eggs. Dr Mosetter believed that it had no effect on blood sugar or insulin. We called it 'friendly sugar'. Some of it, such as the erythritol is said to have the effect of translating fat into energy, rather than what generally happens with sugary excess, namely fructose in overdose, the liver struggles with the overload and turns it into fat. That's the belief of some scientists anyway.

So when you think overdosing on sugar, think bad fat. When American surgeons in Korea compared dead US soldiers with dead Korean soldiers, they observed the plaque-y muck in only the American boys arteries and concluded this was a direct result of fat in the American diet, as Koreans had much less in their diet. They missed the fructose component entirely, and the relation of such sugars to cholesterol, and heart disease. What the cows were fed also was not considered. The idea therefore was the elimination or reduction of animal fats from the diet. This has, in fact occurred across the Western World, but here is the thing: heart disease has not declined much. It isn't the animal fat necessarily, or cholesterol.

It is not the intense taste of modern sugars either that helped escalate the ruin of the American arteries. Ren and colleagues, in *The Journal of Neuroscience* in 2010, experimented with mice by knocking out their taste buds and giving them various foods. Within a few days, the rats began to preferentially eat exclusively from the high-fructose corn syrup supply: their brain centres were hijacked by the chemistry of the sugar, not the taste. Lactose and Galactose are far down on the scale when it comes to perceived sweetness, high-fructose corn syrup is at the top, and this might explain its over-consumption. It is arguably addictive.

It may not just be fattening. Research published in the journal *Injury Prevention* in 2011 suggested that sugar consumption in fizzy drinks was tied to teen violence: it may not be the sugar, but certainly diet plays a role overall in such presentations. US Lawyers have been so convinced of this effect that the so-called 'Twinkie defence' has been used to suggest consumption of junk food has been linked to violence. Jamie Oliver, the celebrity Chef, has gone to schools in the UK and USA and demonstrated that changing what the kids ate altered their challenging behaviour to less troublesome moods and actions.

Those who do abuse refined sugars are generally prone to unhealthy eating; the under-consumption, on the other hand, of *healthy* foods such as fish has been linked to some countries' lower murder and depression rates quite significantly. Fructose and other fat producing substances will combine readily to cause problems that fish oil does not.

So what about fruit? These are packed with sugar, yes, including fructose, but certainly, nature provides us both with sugar as a 'poison', as well as the antidote: fibre. Eating whole fruit will finally put on weight, but not as bad as drinking the juice with the fibre removed. So eat whole fruit, two portions a day, but do not indulge too much. Again, it is about glycaemic load, not index. You would not sit down and eat ten oranges, but squeezed into a glass, the juice without fibre is easy to guzzle, but not healthy or slimming. Fruit juice had in reality NOT been part of our diet until hailstorms damaged citrus crops in California in the Fifties, leading to the production of juiced fruit *en masse*. It caught on.

While we are at it, farmers moved away from Eastern cities in the USA under the Homestead Act, which encouraged the setting up of vast farms in the West. The distances now meant that fresh fruit and vegetables couldn't feed the cities, as they spoiled *en route*. Enter the widespread growing of grains that could be prepped and transported without spoiling, and the American diet had changed forever. Along came corn syrup. Out went healthier food.

Sugar and diabetes are linked of course with studies charting the rise of sugar consumption and diabetes with insulin resistance and its connection to Alzheimer's disease. Rachel Lane and her colleagues at the Mount Sinai School of Medicine have been able to link the genes of Alzheimer's disease with Type II diabetes. This used to be called Adult Onset Diabetes, but since kids increasingly now have it too, the label Type II has stuck. Some experts in 2009 began to call Alzheimer's Type III diabetes because of the common links. Dr Kiyohara and his colleagues, in a 2011 issue of *Neurology*, found the same links. People who did not have diabetes, but who had impaired glucose tolerance were in the same boat, with twice the risk of dementia as those with normal blood sugar levels, and a poor response to carbohydrate with increasing risk. Inflammation is another issue here. Dr Suzanne de la Monte of Rhode Island University has found similar links between brain insulin resistance and two components of Alzheimer's disease, again raising the idea of Type III diabetes.

The recent article in *The Journal of Clinical Investigation* by Dr Steven Arnold has shown the definitive nature of the link between insulin resistance and Alzheimer's. Brain cells have to be re-sensitized to insulin to get them to work again and reduce or reverse cognitive decline.

As I noted, there is now evidence that consuming fructose may hijack brain systems and cause you to eat more. A small preliminary study published in the January 2 2013 issue of the Journal of the

American Medical Association by Kathleen A. Page, M.D., of Yale University and her colleagues conducted a study to examine neurophysiological factors that might underlie associations between fructose consumption and weight gain. They found that there was a significantly greater reduction in hypothalamic cerebral blood flow after glucose vs. fructose ingestion. Dr's Jonathan Purnell and Damien A. Fair of Oregon Health & Science University, Portland, write in an accompanying editorial that these findings support the conceptual framework that when the human brain is exposed to fructose, neurobiological pathways involved in appetite regulation are provoked into increased food intake. Glucose, not fructose, will make you feel full, and slow down your eating.

Simply put, the take-home message is that consumption of refined sugar in today's world is deadly in the quantities we habitually consume by snacking, by 100lbs or more a year.

Now as I mentioned it, it is not sugar alone that is to blame: Deborah Barnes of the VA Medical Centre in San Francisco lists an integrated approach that includes reducing multiple risk factors, which would prevent at least half of the current cases: low education, smoking, physical inactivity, depression, midlife hypertension, diabetes and midlife diabetes. These are all lifestyle issues of course hence the recommendations in her study in the *Lancet Neurology* journal on July 19th 2011.

So although sugar and diet overall are awful, given the role of sugar and diet in the causes above, it is wise to lose the added refined sugar in your diet, or lose much more of your body and brain than you can afford to as you leave your youth behind. Remember, the rot starts early, with your kids, and decades before the signs of damage become apparent.

Here is a tip: substitute the words 'junk food' with the words 'sometimes okay' and you will have a sense of the real value of chocolate and cake and other sources of sugar, fat, death and disability.

Omega 3

Dietary consumption of Omega 3 fatty acids is one of the best studied interactions between food and brain evolution. Docosahexaenoic acid (DHA) is the most abundant Omega 3 fatty acid in cell membranes in the brain, but the human body is not efficient at synthesizing DHA, so we are largely dependent on dietary DHA. It seems likely, as I noted above, that access to DHA during human evolution played a key role in increasing the size of our brains relative to the body. The fact that DHA is an important brain constituent supports the hypothesis that a shore-based diet high in DHA was a prerequisite for growing a bigger brain.

According to Gomez-Pinilla, archaeological evidence shows that early hominids adapted to consuming fish and thus gained access to DHA before this major brain growth occurred. Over the past one hundred years, the intake of saturated fatty acids, linoleic acid and trans- fatty acids has increased dramatically in Western civilizations, whereas the consumption of Omega-3 fatty acids has decreased and hence the Omega 6-3 imbalance. This might explain the elevated incidence of major depression in countries such as the United States and Germany.

It would appear that the addition of Omega 3 into your daily food intake is beneficial. It is not medicine, so taking it daily in food or in supplements is not likely to make you feel better in any real way. However, taking all other areas of brain body optimisation into account, doubtless both benefit from Omega 3 intake in the long run.

It may be that one of the primary effects is simply to keep the Omega 6 balance in place, as the latter is implicated in inflammation, and that at a cellular level is not a good state of affairs. Another implication is for the regulation of blood sugar, as cinnamon does, and as fish oil does too.

The best way to take Omega 3 is via fish consumption. This turns out to be critical, looking at data presented by Gomez-Pinilla, who I mentioned above, writes in the journal *Nature Reviews Neuroscience* in Volume 9 of 2008. Both a country's murder rate and the incidence of depression are linked to the per capita fish consumption.

Omega 3 oil is available from plant sources as well, such as flaxseeds and flaxseed oil (which is quite volatile and needs to be kept cool). However, recent work in *The International Journal of Clinical Practice* is showing that flaxseed is highly interactive with other chemicals such as prescribed medication, as are Echinacea and Yohimbe for instance. Chia, kiwi fruit, butternut and walnuts are also sources of DHA. However, it is much harder for your body to extract the DHA and use it when it has to work on seeds or plant oil rather than fish oil: the fish does the work for us and makes it freely available in its muscle tissue, especially in salmon, cod, sardines, and barramundi. Recall that our mothers used to give us cod liver oil, for good reasons it seems they knew!

Using capsules of fish oil is probably the cheaper and more efficient option, and a wide range are available, most of which have been screened for mercury and other toxins. Most studies look at about

3000mg per day, about three of the common size capsules, and it is good for children as well and there are childhood versions and doses available, usually 500mg. It might lead to thinning of the blood, and might not be a good idea if you are using warfarin or other blood thinners such as aspirin or Ginkgo, so get some pharmacy or medical advice when using it. It seems to have a good effect in attentional issues and in rapid cycling mood disorders as well at higher doses.

As far as our modern brains are concerned, the DHA in Omega 3 oils can affect the function of the synapses, the gaps that allow neurotransmitters in the brain to communicate, as well as cognitive abilities by providing plasma membrane fluidity at synaptic regions. DHA constitutes more than 30% of the total phospholipid composition of plasma membranes in the brain, and thus it is crucial for maintaining the membrane integrity and consequently, brain cell health, according to Gomez-Pinilla. Dietary DHA is needed to maintain the flow of chemicals across the membranes of cell walls, and the function of trans-membrane receptors that support synaptic transmission and cognitive abilities. Omega-3 fatty acids also activate energy-generating metabolic pathways that subsequently affect molecules such as brain-derived neurotrophic factor (BDNF) and insulin-like growth factor 1 (IGF1). IGF1 can be produced in the liver and in skeletal muscle as well as in the brain, and so it can convey peripheral messages to the brain in the context of diet and exercise again confirming the need for an integrated approach to body and brain health.

There is some proof of value in children as well, especially in depression: Nemets and her colleagues, in *The American Journal of Psychiatry* in 2006 found a measured change in levels of depression in a well-controlled study of Omega 3 oils supplements, as they had found in adults in 2002, publishing in the same journal. An NIMH funded double blind trial in teenagers and young adults recently revealed, according to Barbara Cornblatt, the senior researcher, substantial improvements in the majority of the 300 subjects in terms of psychiatric illness and social functioning.

Omega 3, according to the first definitive study, the Bristol University Study of 2011, was found to be significant in the treatment of osteoarthritis in animals.

The February 2012 edition of the journal *Neurology* has a study showing how low levels of Omega 3 affect memory and this is in the context of lower brain volumes in such people.

These are just a few of the proven benefits, including prevention of stroke, improvement in cognitive function, arthritis and blood flow and many more related to Omega 3 consumption.

Some newer preparations such as Ethical Nutrients and Krill oil propose you can take lower doses of oil and still benefit without swallowing a lot of gelatine capsules.

Again, dementia may be a target of fish oils. Researchers at Columbia University looked at a host of nutrients, and discovered higher levels of beta amyloid protein in the blood of those on low fish diets. This is a risk marker, as beta amyloid plaques are part of the plaques and fibrillary tangles found in the brain in Alzheimer's. Fish oil consumption was associated with lower levels, according to Dr Nikolaos Scarmeas: there was no upper limit; eating more and more fish oil meant lower and lower levels of beta amyloid in humans, which improved with higher consumption. Dr Zaldy Tan, in another Neurology journal publication found connections between Omega 3 levels and bigger brains with better test performance.

The preponderance of studies shows Omega 3 to be great for brain and heart function. Not all studies do. Alan Dangour and his colleagues in London looked at a Cochrane Review of Omega 3 and brain and found no correlation. However, as with many studies, they looked at only this single factor, not entire lifestyles which might accompany fish oil or fish consumption. Dangour himself did note that the cognitive benefits might only show up after years of healthy eating, and certainly only in those low in Omega 3 to start, which many in the study were not: they are all healthy adults without any signs of cognitive decline over sixty years old. Which, once again, makes my point: the rot starts early, and secondly, Omega 3 consumption or exercise or pills or anything on its own in isolation might not be the answer we are looking for: we need an integrated approach across the siloes of medicine and healthy behaviour. Dangour and his colleagues did find and recommend the value of increasing fish oil consumption, with the strongest evidence for cardiac health but with enough reasons for brain health as well, especially in those who do feel age encroaching on their brain and body wellbeing. As we saw above, combining fish oil intake is one thing; Tai Chi and movement are another, reducing your sugar and salt intake yet another, covering an integrated body and brain healthy response across the siloes of knowledge.

So think of inflammation, cholesterol being unable to do its job in the presence of inflammation, sugar consumption and Alzheimer's and inflammation, sitting and inflammatory processes, and so on, and you will start thinking like an integrationist. Lifestyle, not just sugar or fish or movement or stress or strain or loneliness alone, but all of the things we do combine to overwhelm our long-living genes. So avoiding inflammation and other cellular issues may explain why coconut oil is looking promising in Alzheimer treatments.

120 years old is not out of the question, but the rot starts early, and it is ALL the things we tend to do that make this look less and less likely, and leave us potentially living the last ten years of our lives in misery.

Salt

Salt intake beyond a point is just not wise, but low sodium levels are also not wise. Given that sodium is present in just about everything we eat today, adding salt would appear to be unwise, as we are likely to get it elsewhere. Salt and stroke, as well as salt and left ventricular muscle mass appear connected in bad ways. Most of the hypertensive, blood pressure raising effect of sodium on Americans and Australians is probably delivered in the bread in their diets, more than adding salt to cooking. You can get the iodine added from fish, so it is not that necessary to add salt to many things.

As for the evidence though, a large Cochrane Review (a really impressive and authoritative review) **could not really find evidence that reducing intake actually increased your lifespan**, despite countless studies that showed a causal link between salt intake and heart disease, and of course blood pressure. It seemed that despite that evidence, reducing intake did not seem to make a difference to longevity overall. The same happened with Omega 3's above. A single causative effect is seldom seen for just one agent added or subtracted from your diet.

A recent review by Professor Rod Taylor at the University of Exeter says that one reason, even in a study of over 6000 people, was that salt reduction alone was insufficient in these studies as well as the fact that a study of over 18 000 people might be necessary before showing any effect. Reducing salt as a single event in the armoury of things to do to save your life is one thing, but not sufficient in itself, all alone in the toolbox: again, the need for integrating this single solution by bundling it with others would seem judicious.

Most doctors and government authorities would still recommend lowering dietary sodium intake. A team of researchers at Case

Western Reserve are finding **some people** are salt sensitive, leading to hypertension as their particular bodies struggle to regulate blood pressure and temperature in the presence of high sodium levels, as published in the journal *Hypertension Research* in April 2011 by Mathew Muller and colleagues. However, even when there is no risk to blood pressure, studies in male twins have found that sodium intake decreases the flexibility of artery walls, published in *The American Journal of Clinical Nutrition* in March 2012 with Viola Vaccarino as an author.

Since average sodium intake by Americans aged two and older is about 3,400 milligrams per day, this is well above the generally recommended cap of 2,300 milligrams per day, or 1,500 milligrams for people older than age fifty or who have high blood pressure, diabetes or chronic kidney disease. Vaccarino's group recommends we all work hard at diminishing our sodium intake as we age. About 80% comes from the processed foods that we eat, not from the source people can most visibly control – the salt shaker. As noted before, bread may be a silent culprit. Again, reducing sodium may only work if other arenas of life are taken care of as well. Reducing your salt while not sleeping well, or while still living under excess stress and leading a sedentary lifestyle just will not help enough. Like fish oil and Tai Chi, it is all part of the picture, not in itself a cure for everything in everyone.

The Mediterranean Diet

Apart from eating a diet strictly made up of food that no human has altered in any way, except by the process of you preparing it, eating food that is clearly identifiable as having once lived is another related option.

The so-called Mediterranean diet (really a lifestyle) is one traditionally followed by people around or near the Mediterranean Sea and is heavy on fish and vegetable consumption, much lighter on land based animal products such as meat or milk. Consisting of a pyramid, with some more typical Western foods seldom eaten at the top, the diet has already been associated with less risk of Mild Cognitive Impairment, which is a precursor in most cases to Alzheimer's or other dementia. MCI may or may not convert to dementia. The diet also serves as helping to avoid the dangers of a high-fat, refined sugar diet, which in research reduces the healthy function of the learning/memory areas of the hippocampus in the brain. See Nikolaos Scarmeas quoted above, and his colleagues in *The Archives of Neurology* 2009 Vol 66, and Molteni and colleagues in *Neuroscience* in 2002, Vol 112(4) respectively. In *The Archives of Neurology*, the so-called *North Manhattan Study* showed in February 2012, in volume 69, that a Mediterranean diet was associated with fewer markers of white matter damage in the brain. A Swedish study done by the *Sahlgrenska Institute* and running for forty years and following thousands of people shows an increased chance of living longer in 20% of those following such a diet, which is more of an eating philosophy than a diet. This evidence, in other related studies, shows the same effects for children as well. And this is in a country with little sunshine! The diet means that people are happy on it, and live longer, healthier lives without restricting much except for portion size. In the USA, plate size has grown from 9" to 12" in a few decades, so portion size in the USA and Australia as well to a lesser extent, is an issue. Mediterranean folk have smaller plates with healthier options, but still enjoy food, bread, wine, love and life... just saying.

Antioxidants/supplements

There is not any compelling research on the value of taking antioxidants as a supplement in pill form. Not only do they not help, but worse, they are clearly harmful.

The evidence comes from no less a publication then *The Journal of the American Medical Association*. By Bjelakovic and colleagues in 2007, this showed that in a study of the data from 232 606 study participants, the use of many antioxidants was lethal. They commented on review that in forty-seven low-bias trials with 180 938 participants, **the antioxidant supplements significantly increased mortality**. After exclusion of selenium trials, beta-carotene, Vitamin A and Vitamin E, singly or combined, significantly increased mortality. Vitamin C and selenium had no significant effect on mortality. One of the issues clearly is the depletion of free radicals at the intracellular level, which removes one of the defences the body has against abnormal cellular formations such as the cancerous ones.

On the other hand, antioxidants in real foods have no such evidence against them. Measuring their Oxygen Radicle Absorbance Capacity (ORAC), prunes, blueberries and blackberries come up trumps compared to tomatoes, zucchini and yellow squash. Cranberries, strawberries, raspberries and pomegranates also do well on the ORAC stakes. Berries, in particular guard against cellular inflammation in the brain and aid signalling by the neurons, according to Barbara Shukitt-Hale and Marshall Miller in the 2012 *Journal of Agricultural and Food Chemistry*.

Worse, in relation to processed antioxidants and dementia, Galasko and colleagues recently found that antioxidants may hasten the cognitive decline in patients with Alzheimer symptoms, publishing in the prestigious *Archives of Neurology* in March 2012.

There is however, some case for micronutrients and health. Studies quoted in Europe, using CO_2 emission machines in crop fields, have shown that the nutrients in vegetables decline markedly as food grows faster in higher levels of carbon dioxide, raising the suspicion that we may not be getting the micronutrients we need, despite eating well. This means that levels of cellular nutrients, especially in peak performers, may not be optimum even when eating well and varied diets in consuming modern vegetables and fruits. Maybe.

Another issue is that traditional blood tests of such nutrients are done by centrifuging the serum out of the blood mixture, ignoring the cells, and thus focusing on the serum content. Cellular analysis by other methods may reveal more about the health of the individual, the same applying to salivary assay of hormones rather than protein-bound hormones in the blood serum. Ask your doctor. However, from my point of view, nutrition first, supplement later, but do so intelligently, and avoid tablet-form antioxidants. Alone, they don't help with ageing, and secondly, they might just kill you off!

Taking supplements, especially antioxidants, is thus a medical science issue, and not an over- the – counter issue. Consult your doctor extensively if you want to go that route. Generally, the doctor will tell you there is little or no evidence that multivitamins are of any use if your diet is healthy and varied, and finally, if the journals are right, they are harmful, coming under the heading: processed food. There has to be a compelling medical argument from your doctor for you to take any supplement in normal daily life.

So who needs vitamins perhaps?

Folate: Pregnant women and those trying to conceive should think of this, and the risk of *spina bifida if they have low levels of* B9.

Vitamin D: People with limited exposure to sunlight such as institutionalised or bedbound elderly, dark-skinned people and veiled women, as well as children or adults who spend a lot of time indoors, in cloudy climates, far from the equator, watch a lot of TV, or whose only exposure is covered by sunblock and clothing, such as religious observant Jews and Muslims. Get your levels checked regularly and opt for the higher ranges. The risk of Multiple Sclerosis increases with distance from the equator.

Vitamin B12: People on a strict vegan diet and the frail aged, who may be eating poorly and or absorbing less from their food, a risk of Vitamin D issues here too.

Others: People on restrictive diets, including those with eating disorders, food allergies or intolerances and those on low-kilojoule weight-loss diets. Supplement depends on the diet so ask your doctor.

Read more: Google: Multivitamins: who needs them, Diet and Fitness Sydney Morning Herald.

Vitamin D

More and more evidence is emerging about the value of vitamin D3 in human health, and in particular, the brain. Adequate levels are challenging to maintain, given the use of sunblock, the migration of Africans to countries where the sun does not really shine, and the growth of conservative religion where women and men are covered by modest clothing. In some cities, large numbers of children are found to be deficient in vitamin D. especially when far from the equator. One in three Australians are, and this is in a country with great weather generally all year round. Worse, if you live your whole life in the south of Australia, in Tasmania, compared to someone who lives far to the North, in Darwin, you will have ten times the risk of Multiple Sclerosis for instance.

This vitamin, a hormone actually, has a wide range of action and deficiency is to be taken seriously... and measured. From just a few thousand a year, now 3 million Australians are being tested. 50% of women in Australia are deficient in spring and during winter, a frightening statistic, and thirty-odd per cent of all of us here are deficient too (see Nowson, *Medical Journal of Australia*, June 2012). Canada is already fortifying food with vitamin D for this reason. However, you can find it in fish liver, fatty fish, mushrooms, milk, soy, and cereal grains as well as fortified foods.

Vitamin D3 has just been found to help clear the damage being laid down in Alzheimer's by Miznicki and colleagues from the University of California, published in *The Journal of Alzheimer's Disease* volume 29, published in 2012.

The Cooper Center Longitudinal Study found that low Vitamin D levels were associated with depressive symptoms, especially in patients with a history of depression, as revealed by Hoang and colleagues in

The Mayo Clinic Proceedings 2011, Vol 86.

Vitamin D deficiency is common in patients with pneumonia who die, and with cancer victims, those with asthma, elderly women who would die without supplementation, and 77% of trauma patients, likewise, are deficient in vitamin D. Fair skinned people may need supplementation, and it boosts the immune system as well. Sportsmen with deficiencies here may suffer more muscle injuries.

Brain, Autism and Vitamin D

There may be a connection in Autism, with some studies correlating the increase in diagnosis with time spent in front of the TV, in other words, indoors. Cannell, in *Medical Hypotheses Vol 70* in 2008, proposed that the apparent increase in the prevalence of autism over the last twenty years corresponds with increasing medical advice to avoid the sun, advice that has probably lowered vitamin D levels and would theoretically lower activated vitamin D (calcitriol) levels in developing brains. Animal data repeatedly showed that severe vitamin D deficiency during gestation deregulates proteins involved in brain development and leads to rat pups with increased brain size and enlarged ventricles, abnormalities similar to those found in autistic children. Children with vitamin D deficient rickets have several autistic markers that apparently disappear with high-dose vitamin D treatment. Oestrogen and testosterone have very different effects on vitamin D's metabolism, differences that may explain the striking male/female sex ratios in autism.

Vitamin D down-regulates production of inflammatory cytokines in the brain, cytokines that have been associated with autism. Consumption of vitamin D containing fish during pregnancy reduces autistic symptoms in offspring. Autism is more common in areas of impaired UVB penetration such as poleward latitudes, urban areas, areas with high air pollution, and areas of high precipitation. Autism is more common in dark-skinned persons and severe maternal vitamin D deficiency is exceptionally common in the dark-skinned.

Breast feeding might not do what it used to do: Shamberger in the Journal of *The American College of Nutrition, in volume 30,* 2011 pointed out that 21st Century women provide virtually no vitamin D in their breast milk, and prenatal vitamin supplementation was necessary with a suggestion that autism might be the risk here.

High dose studies of vitamin D intervention in paediatric autism are currently under way: **Google: Open Label Clinical Trial of Vitamin D in Children with Autism ClinicalTrials.gov**

Anecdotal evidence is showing that Africans who have fled regional instability for sanctuary in Scandinavia might for the first time be showing increased autism in their ranks; and dementia. Swedish scholars are now exploring why there is an increased incidence of Autism in Somalian children in Sweden. That is compared to their cousins at home who are virtually free of the condition, or at least reported in lower volumes.

See **The Swedish Local Swedish researchers explore Somali-autism link.** More troubling is that 12% of the children diagnosed with Autism in Minneapolis reported that their home language was Somalian, even though they made up only 17% of the entire community. That was worrying, and drew attention to the MMR vaccines, which nowhere else have been shown to be dangerous. Minneapolis, as you may know, is not known for its stunning sunlight hours during the year.

It may not be only the young with this issue: as we age, it becomes harder to synthesize our own vitamin D from sunlight alone, so we need to be mindful and have our levels checked. Given the risks, it might be a good idea for all to be checked. In July 2009, *The Journal of Alzheimer's Disease* began to report early studies at the David Geffen School of Medicine at UCLA that vitamin D and synthetic compounds derived from naturally occurring curry spice, turmeric-curcumin, showed promise in clearing the amyloid plaques in the brain of victims of Alzheimer's.

Another issue with autism and stomach bacteria may be an issue. Overgrowth of clostridia, treated with vancomycin, actually seems to improve symptoms. However, these kids cannot live on the stuff, so more research is needed.

Carbs

Yes. Finally. The big C. Simply put, sure, we do not really need carbs. We can live quite happily, sort of, with only protein and fat, and manufacture our own carbs. However, when we do that, we produce cortisol. Remember cortisol? Pro-inflammatory cortisol, which we produce as a stress hormone, which means less sex hormones? We also know that diets such as the Atkinson Diet got some bad press about kidneys and things. So carbs, as we consider them, namely vegetable-derived, never hurt anyone, and it is easy to extract the energy from them direct to muscle and brain. Most importantly, people on low carb diets get really ratty and irritable, so do not eliminate them from your diet, unless they are processed carbs, which really, if you read above, are not on.

The Rules:

So by now, I guess you are thoroughly confused, or miserable. So here are some rules to follow, just to be sure:

1. Follow a Mediterranean Diet, or a low human interference diet for overall brain and body health.

2. Make sure you drink half your body weight in water ounces each day, or 300-350ml per ten kilograms, male-female.

3. Consume three portions of fatty fish, e.g. grilled salmon each week, or at least 3000mg of good quality fish oil each day, including Krill oil if possible.

4. Avoid antioxidant supplements, and eat a diet with lots of dark berries, especially blueberries, for instance, some red wine, dark chocolate and other natural flavonoid filled fruit or cocoa sourced food.

5. Drink coffee and tea in moderation, without milk or sugar if possible.

6. Avoid excess sugar and salt intake, and processed fruit products, including fruit juices. Avoid dairy and grains, but watch your calcium young women!

7. Supplement your diet with Vitamin D after assessment, Vitamin B complex, and perhaps magnesium, Co enzyme Q10 especially if on Statin drugs, and perhaps Selenium, and Vitamin C when necessary for a cold or influenza. Get medical advice.

8. Avoid excess alcohol, which is fermented from sugar.

9. Eat breakfast cereals and bread if you must, with 99-100% whole grains, not less, and not processed; add some cinnamon and honey for taste.

10. Eat food that is a fresh and organic as possible: frozen fruit and vegetables may be good enough. Eating grass fed meat may also be fine.

Oh yeah, and move closer to the equator!

Super Foods

My colleagues at Core Performance in the USA have set out a list of superfoods. These can be found at the website at **Google: Core Performance.com superfoods.html**. Many of these are largely commonly sourced in the USA, but you can get them if you hunt around in other countries as well.

Jack adjusted his food intake following the rules above. He gradually lost weight and felt better and better about himself, losing about 500gms a week until seventy-eight kgs was achieved. This, he felt, was close enough to seventy-six kg, his goal weight.

So now you know enough to change your life and your brain and body health significantly, right?

Sadly NO. Few of you reading this will do much at all, except get really depressed, tell your friends how you read this book and decided you were just going to die anyway, and that nothing can be done because you have no choice but to sit and eat and die young. This Guru bloke from Australia has pointed out you lead a toxic existence and the whole world would have to change in order for you to manage your health better. I mean everything, but everything is going to kill you, and you would have to make MASSIVE changes to get healthy.

Nothing could be further from the truth. Little things make a huge difference. But here is the thing about change, as Mel Robbins says: you are NEVER going to feel like it. You have to force yourself to engage in the process of change.

But yes, I agree. It seems too daunting when you consider the changes you might choose to make or have to make: it is not. I am not a guru, nor the expert on how you change.

There is a way out. Read on to find out how change is easier, change on your own terms. Change where you do not have to force yourself too much. You just have to become the expert on what exactly makes you change.

Something Extra from Gomez-Pinilla: Brain Foods

When it comes to nutrients that affect cognitive function, here are some more:

Curcumin: contained in Turmeric, the spice in curry, this has been found to ameliorate cognitive decline in models of Alzheimer's and Traumatic Brain Injury in rats. Small wonder Alzheimer's is pretty rare in India, where the British introduced curry to mask the rotten meat they brought. Vitamin D compounds in the spices may explain the effect. Also, the low, low BMI of most rural Indians is a factor too.

Flavonoids: These are found in cocoa, tea, ginkgo, citrus fruit, wine (especially red), and dark chocolate among other things. Combining flavonoids with exercise in animal models has shown improvement in cognition in the young, and elderly alike. Drinking bottles of resveratrol is not the same thing, so it is not wise to do that either.

Saturated Fat: Yes, you heard me. Except this promotes cognitive decline in animal models, aggravates cognitive impairment after brain injury, and exacerbates cognitive decline in the elderly human too. Butter, ghee, suet, lard, coconut oil, cottonseed oil, palm kernel oil, cream, cheese and meat are all culprits to be limited in consumption. And if you are Ashkenazi Jewish, then lay off meat pretty much totally, down to one or less times a week. But, this is from one authority: there are others who stress the need for saturated fat. So what do you do? Integrate everything into one healthy lifestyle, and hope for the best.

Vitamins: B6, B12 or B9 folate has positive effects on memory performance in women across the age spectrum, and B12 in animal models improves cognition in those fed on low choline diets. Vitamin E does help in animal models after traumatic brain injury, and reduces cognitive decline in the elderly as well. Keep the JAMA studies in mind though when it comes to antioxidants in pill form, although combinations of C, E and carotene delay cognitive decline in the elderly, but may hurt otherwise.

Choline: Found in egg yolks, soy, beef, chicken, veal, turkey, liver and lettuce, this could be useful according to animal models of post-seizure repair, and there is a causal link between cognition in animals and humans and choline. Reducing acetyl cholinesterase by tablet, in other words, increasing the availability of acetylcholine is in effect a delaying treatment in Alzheimer's. So is coconut oil, advised against here. Go figure…

Calcium, Zinc, Selenium: Lifelong low selenium is correlated with lower cognitive function in humans, and high levels of calcium and zinc are thought to co-exist with a faster decline in the elderly.

Zinc is to be avoided in such adults, and is contained in oysters, a small amount in beans, nuts, almonds, whole grains, and sunflower seeds. Calcium of course is found in milk and other places. Selenium is thought to be beneficial, so consume it in nuts, cereals, meat, fish and eggs. Zinc and copper are necessary for mental health though...

Copper/Iron: While many quacks might want to eliminate metals, Copper is essential and cognitive decline in Alzheimer's correlates with low plasma concentrations of copper. Copper is found in oysters, beef/lamb liver, Brazil nuts, blackstrap molasses, cocoa and black pepper. Iron treatment normalizes cognitive function in young women, and higher rather than low limit levels of ferritin are essential in athletes for optimal oxygen transport. Zinc may be implicated in depression, and in the inflammatory response related to albumin transport of zinc in the blood. Too little zinc may thus also be a cause of problems, as suggested by Dr James Greenblatt in his book *The Breakthrough Depression Solution*, published by Sunrise River Press in 2011 and reviewed on my website under recommended reading.

A parting word from Gomez-Pinilla. A longitudinal study included more than one hundred years of records in 300 Swedish families. An individual's risk for diabetes and early death was increased if their paternal grandparents grew up in a time of food abundance rather than times of shortages. The BDNF system is particularly sensitive to epigenetic modifications that influence cognitive functions that clearly can be transmitted across generations. Diet will influence genetic events in your offspring long after you have gone. The rot not only starts early, it may have started for you before you were born, and will affect your offspring when you have gone; so be the first generation that is moderate in lifestyle. For those of us who have children, making sure they are not spoiled by huge abundance is vital now more than ever. Eat well, but healthily. Start now.

Chapter Four

green

motivating change; you are the expert on you!

ndrew was always doing some kind of gym stuff. The problem was, like three-quarters of the people in most big cities, he would sign up for gym in January, and seldom go. His personal trainer was his favourite Drill Sergeant person in the world, but occasional injury to his shoulder and lower back seemed to get in the way just as he was getting somewhere. Holidays, pressure at work, the twins starting school, his wife's new job requiring she travel. All of these contributed to his serial failures at sustaining his fitness levels. "Exercise is vital to me," he would often say, "but there is just no time, something always gets in the way". Like most people, he aspired to get to the gym, but only managed this in fits and starts. He put on a kilogram a year, and finally was diagnosed with rising cholesterol and blood sugar. Scared witless by his doctor's dire warnings, and with a young family, he went straight to the gym and registered for a two-year contract. After twelve weeks, he cancelled the contract and incurred a penalty: "I just could not get there; but I

know my brain and body are just not working, I have to DO something".
But he does nothing.

Most of us would recognize Andrew's predicament: most people
who sign up to a health club do not sustain it or seldom go, or find they
run on 'deficit time' in their day to day existence, and so do not get
fit or stay fit. One of the problems can be that this is not fun for most
people, which explains why Zumba and other health crazes take off so
well, as they provide novelty and social interaction for a longer period.

The problem in getting to a health centre, is in reality, the same as
the food dilemma – convenience. Prepared food is a solution for the
busy adult and so yummy for the kid or adolescent, but it is killing
us. Fast food is a solution to time constraints imposed by modern
life, and so is being unfit. We cannot find the time in a busy day,
hence the rise of twenty-four-hour gyms. A second problem has
been the reliance on trainers who are still immersed in isolating,
body muscle building, which has risks of injury and boredom.
Another attraction of the twenty-four-hour gym is the absence of
sales staff. Using the available Tablets, more people sign up than
would be the case when confronted by sales teams: this is because
we trust a computer-tablet to not have a convincing and coercive
sales pitch that drives us to do stuff we should not really want to
do. We usually do not trust people in those environments, and we
also fail to trust ourselves. When you touch on the tablet screen to
commit, it is on your terms, or so you think.

So now you know about the absolute value of food and movement
management. You simply HAVE TO eat healthily and move more. So
why, knowing this, do you continue to do NEITHER?

The problem may be in the words 'HAVE TO': Senge writes in
The Fifth Discipline that people do not mind changing, but they hate

to be told they have to change. Doing things for your own reasons, on your own terms, is more tolerable.

CHANGE on your own terms: this is the issue. Modern lifestyles are difficult to change. It is hard to find time to cook and move in healthy ways when we live on deficit time. Deficit sleep means we do not feel like getting up and losing sleep to head to the gym, jog, or cycle. Deficit time means we wake up at the last possible moment, hit the snooze button (not a good thing to do as you will see later), dash around under vanishing time, and spend the day chasing our tails and deadlines, which really make eating well and moving effectively pretty awesome challenges.

Change, real, meaningful, lasting change to our lifestyles is thus hard to accomplish, not impossible, in fact, quite simple really but most people find deficit time management hard to achieve.

Change itself is scary, as any change is interpreted by the non-conscious brain as novel, as effortful or risky to the organism. The need for change has to be quite compelling to warrant the effort, and of course, the threat of sacrifice.

Motivation 101:
Change = Sacrifice, and successful change is sacrifice on your own terms.

Let us imagine Andrew struggling to change. He is at Point A in his life, and he is aware, or certainly with his doctor's help, becoming increasingly aware and scared that there is a better version of him out there somewhere. Let's name that Point B. He looks up from where he is now body and brain-wise, at Point A, and he sees the Holy Land, Point B, where he is a magnificent specimen of forty-five-year-old manhood.

Even for Andrew, the thought of attempting to move toward the desired heaven of Point B was NOT attractive. The distance he perceived between Point A and Point B was miles too far. He had TRIED several dozen times to get to Point B sustainably, but had failed each time in some way. So the D for distance between Point A and Point B was a function of his experience, and the negative defensive emotion that rose in his chest when he contemplated what it might take to get to the holy grail of Point B was demotivating: "It's all too hard" is what he told me. Sacrifice for no advantage is not worth it, reasonably.

Instead of motivating him to get off his butt and get moving and eating well, the realization of what he had failed to do in the past and what threats now faced him, because of his prior failures, created a huge ambivalent barrier of emotion in him: "On the one hand, I want it, but on the other hand, it is too hard to get. The sacrifice will be for nothing: I will fail again as I have before, all effort, and no reward". His view of reality is that he was going to get old and die earlier, and there was nothing that he could do to avoid this dreadful fate. Nothing HE COULD DO. He felt a distinct lack of self-efficacy, no sense that anything in his power to do would or could make a difference to the inevitable, and so he became resigned to that apparent fact. His helplessness, despite his desire to change.

Change is particularly hard for just that reason. Human resolve to change is a tricky thing. People do not mind changing, as Senge has noted, but changing because you have to is harder than it looks on the surface. Motivation from another source is limited compared to motivation that comes from somewhere deeply personal inside your head. Extrinsic motivation is being paid to do something, or being ordered to do something, which is fine if you are engaging in some concrete task, but it does not work for things you should do for the sake of it, for the love of it, or because it might be good for you in some way. Intrinsic motivation means that you have found your purpose in doing something, for the love of it, for the sake of becoming better in some meaningful way, not as a way of avoiding death or disability when nothing you seem to have done changed that destiny. Learned helplessness is awful, and in extremes, it can be deadly.

You would think a diabetic would take their medication readily given the huge risks if they do not, but they often struggle to keep their blood sugar as tightly regulated as they should. People who get drunk and beat up their partners in a marriage usually lose out, but they do not stop drinking. People who bite their nails struggle for a lifetime to stop in some cases. People with memory issues can cope well with a digital diary, but tend not to use them regularly, or lose them. Smokers know that one in two will die from it, but they continue.

Change, real, meaningful change, is difficult to accomplish. Enduring change is hard. Think about how long it took you to get to the gym, stick to a diet, be on time at appointments, stop biting your nails, review your life insurance, give up smoking or sugar in coffee, and so on. For most, it can take two years of thinking about it. Even when people reach their goal, e.g. their goal weight, slipping back into old patterns is more common than staying with the new behaviour, if the emotional drivers are incorrect, or more clearly, wrong for you.

Why is change so hard, is it just the sacrifice? The loss of resolve after successive failures with no results? Will power? Perseverance? Intrinsic vs. Extrinsic Reward?

Reward: the way the brain works on reward is related to a chemical called dopamine. It is not necessarily the rewarding results of success that stimulate dopamine, but the EXPECTATION of reward that triggers this very old system in the brain. The expectation that if I do something, I will achieve something directly because of it, is dopamine's role.

Think of a cocaine addict who gives up the habit: just the sight of a credit card or rolled banknote or mirror or some white powder will trigger a craving; for craving, read: expectation of reward. In smokers for instance, the withdrawal from the previous cigarette triggers an expectation that the next cigarette will remove the uncomfortable feeling that abstinence produces. This expectation drives the next light-up, so that the 'pleasure' is not dopamine, but the reduction of the discomfort of withdrawal. The dopamine tells you to expect the reduction in the pain of withdrawal, or tells you that you have to have more of the heroin, and nothing else will feel as good – expectation of reward. This is so strong that even though the effects of the first use of heroin are never to be repeated, the addict will keep on trying for a lifetime until they die to get even close to that first ebullient reward, without ever managing it, so strong is the expectation that they will, if they just try.

A healthy lifestyle should become equally addictive. It should become something we adopt. However, it is hard indeed.

If you know that doing something will definitely bring pleasure, and instant pleasure, the chances are that you will pursue it strongly. So a heroin addict has trained their brain from the first hit that doing it again will reliably produce a huge rush of pleasure, so they seek it out, despite the knowledge that this will never happen. But they fool themselves, and anyway, the pain of withdrawal is SO nasty. They keep on using just enough, a few $10 bags a day, to avoid the loss of expectation of reward, a painful withdrawal.

A healthy lifestyle is more elusive, more subtle and esoteric in producing delayed and incremental reward, and requires ongoing commitment, unlike a drug or other thing we can do, which gives immediate reward, and we expect it to. There is some elusive quality we need to inspire in ourselves to drive our resolve to change over time. We have to find that behaviour addictive, and want to adopt it, rather than comply with some doctor's or spouse's wishes.

Andrew was required by his doctor to comply with medical advice, but he did not. Andrew would need to ADOPT a range of behaviours for his own good reasons to succeed, but he failed in that too. Like many, he failed to comply for long enough. Adopting such healthier behaviours for his personally-derived good reasons, rather than the doctor's demands, would have created an ongoing success story.

Smoking

A great example here is smoking. The gases from a cigarette are hardly attractive. They are smelly, toxic, expensive and dangerous. Where is the reward? Nowhere actually, in the act of smoking itself, except for one thing: each cigarette rewards you by overturning the painful withdrawal from the previous cigarette. The pleasure you feel is actually the disappearance of the discomfort that arises when you stop smoking, which then disappears when you light up. Secondly, given no immediate fatal cause-and-effect, you may need to smoke perhaps 300 000 times until you become aware that cigarette = danger, so the brain does not get scared, until the doctor says, "Oh-oh!" Then it is too late. So the drivers to stop are buried deeply in us, despite the smell and cough, etc.

There may be rewards in our society that support smoking, such as in advertising, or in social reward, which may not make sense to us.

Melanie Laurent, a thirty year old Jewish-French actor famous for her cinematic roles which often support her third generation Holocaust survivor status, and commonly this generation goes into creative arts, is also famous for a video interview of herself in black and white, without makeup, and smoking throughout. Half way through, a small cough alerts us to tarry phlegm in her lungs. Typically, her cigarette lands up having a long, limp ash dangling from it, as she talks animatedly, with an earthy voice typical of blue packet French smokes. Shocked? No makeup, smoking, hair messy? Yet this video is accredited with having brought her work from overseas directors and producers, a few years back. The image of this sexy young talent is redolent with the stereotypes of past advertising when smoking was glamorous, and harkens us back to Breakfast at Tiffany's, or James Dean. The French have the tightest public smoking laws in the world, happily ignored by most locals there, often smoking metres from the gendarmerie in restricted areas. Laurent's insouciance about her appearance resonates with us, she epitomizes a natural, carefree gal, still beautiful no matter what she is wearing or doing at the time, not concerned with what people might think. This is rewarded. Her French diet and lifestyle may protect her for now, but 66 000 smoking-related deaths a year are reported in France, 6 000 more from passive smoking, and the deaths will increase over the next decades, declining in men, but increasing in women unfortunately. One in eight French deaths each year is cigarette-related. The 300 000 cigarettes start the death cycle one light up at a time, ageing you slowly, and the rot, which starts early, may still be encouraged by youthful irreverence for old age. In smokers, old age comes early. Curious as it may be for us to love this young woman for her beauty and saucy, sexy attitude supported by rewards of work and a feeling of rebellion, still, one in two smokers, half of all of them, will die from smoking-related ill health. Ms Laurent knows them too, but...?

As for any unhealthy behaviour, for her to give up a life threatening but not immediately dangerous lifestyle practice will require the welling up in her of a particular quality which drives change, namely an intrinsic motivator, such as a pregnancy perhaps. Not a compelling speech from her family or friends, but a warm, supportive relationship, which allows her to be herself, but stirs in her a self-derived desire to change something extrinsically rewarded in her life and career, but dangerous to something she might cherish more.

Models of Motivation to Healthy Change: Self-efficacy

Is there an intrinsic quality that will drive you to follow the movement and nutrition recommendations in the first chapters here? Are there models of change in such areas, which can be helpful to help engage and retain us in healthy behavior, and inspire intrinsic motivation?

Katherine Thirlaway and Dominic Upton have conducted serious reviews of the various models of change in their book *The Psychology of Lifestyle*: Promoting health behaviour, published by Routledge in 2009 (you can read a review from a link in my website **http://www.roysugarman.com/recommended-reading**) if you are interested in the various models.

One factor continuously emerges from their analysis of the models however, common to all of them: the concept of self-efficacy which I mentioned above.

First put forward by Albert Bandura decades ago, this refers to a belief that one is actually capable of behaving in a way to attain a specified, cherished set of goals. Our personalized belief systems around this foundation, namely that we can make a difference by behaving in a certain way toward a powerfully desired end goal, will profoundly affect our resolve to change and our relationships with others.

Self-efficacy means you have a belief that what you will do and can do must make a real difference, and you honestly believe that your cherished goals are attainable, and what you are doing or setting out to do will reach the desired outcome. Fostering that belief is the goal of motivational experts.

In this regard, Sheldon Williams and his colleagues have written that someone who attempts to weave a spell of inspired speech around you will not have nearly the same success compared to You coming up with your own web of inspiring speech, a speech containing your personal, valid reasons for change in the pursuit of cherished goals, not someone else's. So an inspiring dietician or personal trainer, filling your head with all kinds of sweet or punishing talk is only visiting the life you are living, and so is not going to have ultimate control over what you finally do. Not for long.

This defines then the difference between compliance with someone else's demands on you, and you adopting healthy behaviour change for your own reasons. As Williams et al note, in their book *"Self-determination theory in the clinic; motivating physical and mental health"* published by Yale University Press in 2003, reviewed on my website, a **warm relationshi**p with a person you relate to is more likely to get you to be motivated by what they are saying, than by the content of what they are saying. Liking the motivating person who is trying to get you to change is important; warm supportive relationships are useful, but not enough. You, in this regard are the expert in You:

- You are the expert in how you have failed in the past.

- You are the expert in how you have succeeded in the past.

- You are the expert in the reasons you might want to change.

- You are the expert in what arguments work to inspire you.

- You alone know what sacrifices to make and when you feel ambivalent about them.

- You alone know the thoughts and doubts in your head.

- You alone know who around you is best able to help or hinder your attempts at goals.

- You alone know why a particular goal is important to you.

- You alone make the most compelling arguments to change yourself.

- You only feel great when you are responsible for the direction your life is going.

- You alone feel great when you get better and better at doing what is important to you.

- You alone are living your life, uniquely. Others do not really know you that well.

- You alone are inspired by your purpose in life, if you can find it.

Autonomy, Mastery and Purpose

Considering the bullet points above, you might see three powerful concepts emerging, as explained by people such as Dan Pink when he reviewed the surprising components of what drives us to change or face creative challenges in the 21st Century.

Let us imagine I pay you to take a health test, and I pay you to take on healthy behaviour. This would work, right? Not so much. What if I pay for your health club? *Nada.*

Employers in the USA, faced with paying huge and increasing amounts for employee health care cover (the USA spends more than four times as much per head of population than any country that has universal free healthcare, and the USA does not have this), wanted their workers to do a simple online Health Risk Assessment, taking about fifteen minutes or so to complete. Even giving each of them a $100 or $150 incentive to spend seldom engaged more than 10% of them to do this, if the presentations I have attended at the Disability Management Employers Coalition meetings and the Wellness Councils of America (WELCOA) literature are anything to go by. People who did the HRA and pocketed the incentive then failed to follow up and mitigate their health risks, as they expected to be paid, and their motivation to change their health had not been boosted at all. Nine out of ten such schemes by employers fail, according to WELCOA. Given the data they collect, few employers actually use this data to do anything effective to enhance the health of their employees. The model is often wrong, not based on self-efficacy.

If your teenagers do not clean up their room, paying them to do so means they will do it because you are paying, and if you stop, they stop. Simple, and you can accept that. Screaming and nagging may only work so far. However, let us say they want to take a gap year overseas in ten months' time. Now you can use that to say, ok, MY cherished goal is that you should clean up your room. Do it every week for the next forty weeks and I will give you $20 a week as part of your pocket money, which will give you $800 towards it, or something similar. The kid has a goal, you have a goal, that coincides, and so now you stand a chance, as the intrinsic goal of overseas dominates the child, not the money as such, and not in compliance with your own wishes. No goal, and the kid will leave the room dirty and forego the money if cleaning up has no overseas goal attached; otherwise, it goes into the too hard basket.

As Dan Pink has pointed out (see his humorous presentation of his book and related work at **www.Ted.com**), paying people to do things which they should do for the sake of doing it, because it is the right thing to do, or for the sheer enjoyment of it, reduces their motivation to do that act, which is rather surprising. Think of professional sportsmen in that context who used to play for fun and the feeling of advancement of skill.

It turns out that if you want to get people to adopt healthy behaviour change, pure financial rewards are not only ineffective, but might have the opposite effect. If we take money off the table, then more intrinsic motivators are required: things that are vitally important to us matter more than others, or what is important to others.

So for instance there is no research showing that wearing a pedometer engages men or women in healthy behaviour change across time. However, one study in women shows it did work, but only when part of a highly integrated programme, not a standalone 10 000 step programme.

So we get to the three principles driving change that I listed above.

Autonomy: what is important, vitally important to me

Vitally inherent in us is the desire to chart our own existence, to navigate life according to our own wishes. We wish to direct where we go and remove uncertainty from our future. This is in essence a form of self-efficacy, in and of itself. The desire to see that what we want out of life is attainable. The desire to control the life we are experiencing, on our own terms. We want to captain our ship, master our destiny; this is what we most desire. And, from self-determination theory, this revolves around what is vitally important to us.

Although many experts tout self-esteem as a key predictor of bad or good outcomes, there is no real body of scientific evidence to confirm this. Self-efficacy, yes, self-esteem, no. Low self-esteem may actually direct many people to become determined to make the world sit up and take notice, and so may work as a motivator, but it does not predict disaster. The world is full of successful people who think they were just lucky, that they did not deserve success.

So self-efficacy fits into the desire to seek and succeed in the outcomes we most want, by changing behaviours in the here and now that have the biggest chance of turning out well in the future, around essential purposes in our lives. In this way, autonomy is entirely in sync with and driven by our frontal-executive areas in the brain, areas which make decisions for us and drive our goals for the future, as well as the best actions to take now to ensure the most advantageous outcomes for us at some distant point in time.

A person's autonomy should never be disrespected, but so many situations exist when it is ignored by others, and this does not support the person in healthy behavioural change. On the other hand, showing respect for someone's autonomy does help support change. This allows a sense of relatedness for the person who is struggling to change, knowing their desire to go in a certain direction is supported by and is meaningful to others.

Autonomy and the desire to preserve it around vital issues for us, have a strange side effect, something explained by attribution theory.

Fundamental Attribution Error: It is not me, it is YOU.

Attribution theory concerns itself with how we make judgements about our own and other people's behaviour. Behaviour is typically explained in terms of either internal or external events in someone's life. The side effect of this is that we tend to over-emphasize internal events to explain other people's behaviour, and on external events to excuse our own. So if HE is nasty, that is because he has a rotten personality, but if I am, that is because, well, er... I am stressed at this time. This comes naturally to us.

In other words, if I fail to engage in healthy behaviours because lifestyle events are beyond my autonomous control, other people are likely to view me as weak. Employers, hoping to engage me as a worker in their wellness programs will see my failure to use them as weak, lazy, obstinate, distrusting, frustrating, and label me a couch potato and incorrigible. On the other hand, they might ignore the demotivating effect of the medicalized nature of the online programs, the negative messages they propose, the out of touch weekly updates for pregnancy or cancer week or smoking cessation or other topics which are irrelevant to me, or my gender, or my age. They may ignore the fact I do not believe that sitting in front of a computer is healthy: nor do I need to earn twenty million compliance points in two years of hard work, which buys me a pair of running shoes, I hate running anyway, and points achieve nothing more meaningful in reward terms.

In another variance of this fundamental attribution error, if I do something healthy in terms of changing my behaviour, under the guidance of a program or person, I will attribute my success to my hard work, and discount the input of the outside systems. However, the people who create these systems will see my success as emerging from the use of their system, not my perseverance and hard work. Worse, if I see them as the source of my success, then I own no success of my own at all and it should cease when I disengage.

Wow. However, that is human nature for you. We own our successes, distance our failures and ascribe them to outside circumstances; that is how we 'roll.'

So motivation to change depends on how supported we feel in guiding our own lives.

We can do what is important to us, uniquely to us, and perhaps no other. And when we find that, we need to get better and better at it, to sustain our sense that it is all worth it at the end of the day.

Mastery: Growth is progress.

Three out of four people who join a gym or health club or fitness centre never make the most of it. Most will leave within the first twelve weeks. One of the reasons is that the trainer we work with knows something we do not know: most people do not fully experience the benefits of training for a few hours a week within that short period of time. Only after three months will we usually see things changing: there is no quick fix. Perseverance will only pay off if the trainer can stimulate and engage us in what is improving – with regular changes of pace and challenge and frequent feedback and proof of how we are doing compared to where we started. Measuring our successes in real terms will help us manage that period better.

Another issue perhaps is we do not really need to bench press anything in real life, unless we live on the San Andreas Fault, and even then, trying to bench-press your collapsed building off you is unlikely to help. Bench pressing is only useful in a bar after a few drinks, and you can boast: if this is your goal, fine, then the principle of mastery will apply.

Mastery implies that we get better and better at doing what is important to us. Not others but us; it is related to autonomy. We have to discover what is vitally important to us, a cherished goal as step one, and then get better and better at doing what is meaningful to us, step two, and this may be unique to everyone.

Mastery implies that we exceed our own self-image on a regular basis. This means overcoming both setbacks and gratuitous advancement (luck) and staying focussed on who we are, and how we get better and better at being who we are when we are at our best.

A doctor who points out that our high cholesterol or smoking is killing us is not really taking into account the idea of mastery: taking a pill, how does that sustain us in getting better and better at what might be important to us? Compliance with the doctor and medication depends on this fitting in with where we want to go in life and how that will unfold in terms of personal growth. Being told to do something, no matter how advisable, is not motivating.

So a wellness program at our workplace or provided by our HMO cannot, by definition, be personalized to what we regard as important or what is meaningful to us in order to and help us reach our goals. Another aspect is that we may not see ourselves as lacking wellness if we see it as disease, after all, we are not sick as we perceive it, so why engage with a wellness programme? Where is the immediate reward that we are highly wired to achieve?

Vick decided he wanted to leave his job, to make more money. But every time he thought of it, he went cold in the stomach and chickened out. He came to see me for brain assessment as he felt he needed insight. I saw that his negative emotions were just fine, quick and accurate perception of the threats he faced, and of his perception of not slowing down, which would have suggested a problem. However, the positive emotion perception was way out of whack, to use a technical term. Working with him, we established his goal was to make money, but he had never focused on what he wanted to do with the money, why this was important. It turns out his cherished goal was to act on stage, but he could never make money that way. Really, what he wanted was power to change the world, using money. He then realised that money would buy him the influence to move in the circles that lead to political life, and there he could both act, and wield power, using the contacts he made in moneyed circles. This vision spurred him on and he moved on to live his dream, having found his purpose, and change the world for the better. I would vote for him. His wife would not: she folded her tents and left him, unable to sustain the relationship in the face of the essential changes he was making. This loss of his relationship took the wind out of his sails and he sat around for a month doing nothing, mired in a fog again. When he went back to his goal sheet, he reworked it after three years and it mobilized his executive functions, he forged ahead again, revitalized by the expectation of new rewards and the desire to un-focus from his failed marriage.

Purpose:

Finding a sense of purpose means you have activated your resolve to change. People with a purpose in life accept change as inevitable and interpret their anxiety as excitement. This gives them an edge. Relatedness is another concept that is similar in kind to this. A purpose that is greater than the self tends to have longer legs on life's journey. 'Meaning', via relatedness of a greater purpose, allows soldiers to die willingly for a cause. The critical aspect is to focus your efforts around a single, defining entity in your self-image; for instance, if a psychiatrist, to aspire to improve the treatments just a fraction, or if an artist, to advance the cause of fine art with each work. Purpose is a definition of intent, a focus to each desire you have, so that random needs or wants do not derail you from your life's work. And your life's work is defined by a moving target, your self-image.

Vick found that for selfish reasons he lacked courage, until he saw himself waving to his constituents, loved by thousands for leading them to a better life. Then he jumped ship and swam for success. In doing so, he changed as a person, and widened the gap between him and his partner, which had begun when he had started to grow out of their childhood sweetheart relationship, and she had not.

He is not alone in experiencing such changes.

I recall Philippa well. She came to see me, determined to do something she had never done. Lose eighteen lbs. She was getting married at thirty years old, fulfilling a dream. She had her wedding dress made, ordering it from China, but several sizes too small. She watched her mother's face fall to the floor when it arrived. Her mother nearly cried at the fact that she would never see her daughter wear it. Philippa's cherished dream was to wear this dream dress and look awesome in it, something so unachievable her dietician thought she was psychotic and would die if she tried. Philippa was barely four-foot ten in height and eighteen pounds was massive loss for her. Only the Chinese make wedding dresses that small. So Philippa came to me to find out if I thought she was crazy, and to convince her to forget it. I said, okay, let's do this. We explored why this goal was so cherished. A lonely child, Philippa played with Barbie and Ken Dolls and all her fantasies of love and life centred on these slim, perfect figures. When her time came, she wanted nothing less. She had no idea why this cherished belief was so important to her though. Her emotions in relation to her wedding were those of a four or five year old child, not a mature woman. Her agony reached back twenty-five years, and was only going to be assuaged by losing a massive percentage of her body. Searching for meaning and asking her to explain more and more of this cherished goal, diving deeper, she responded finally that the dolls' lives were controlled by her, a greater force, and this made her life predictable: if only she were thin, he would never leave her. Thin meant forever. Thin meant some invisible force outside would grab him by the waist and force him to be with her. It took her fiancé a long time to explain to her why his cherished goal was never to leave her, why his life direction was the invisible force that would hold him to her. In her heart she knew the weight was not the issue, but that was all she could think of to work her sense of self-efficacy around. She lost eleven pounds, a sterling achievement, and a nice lady with a sewing machine and two panels of lacy material did the rest. I thought she looked lovely. So did her Ken. And no one could see the eight inch platforms under the new lace that boosted her to five foot six. Raise high the roof beams, carpenters, indeed. Her self-image moved to where it should have been all the time.

You can tell when people have found their purpose that fits with their self-image: they use a kind of language to let you know. The founding fathers of motivational engineering, Bill Miller and Steve Rollnick called this style of talking 'Change-Talk', as opposed to 'Sustain-Talk' as mentioned above.

Change talk sounds like DARN-C. The letters in it stand for Desire, Ability, Reason, Need, and finally, Commitment. When you listen, you hear people express the desire for change, and they know what they really need, what is important to them, the cherished goal, the overarching purpose. They need to express that well in their desire to change.

You will hear them enumerate the strengths they have, the ability to change that will propel them forward.

They clearly state the reasons why changes are imperative for them, how these reasons stack up to a cherished goal. There are compelling needs around their self-image that will be fulfilled, reasons why change will change their lives for the better, and there is a clarity to that. Moreover, there is a single, defining element to all the changes they want to make, related to things beyond just their paltry desires. This is their image of their deep self.

Finally, they can begin to see that DARN-C supports them in changing on their own terms: so their commitment is there and this goes down in writing for most part, like a contract for a health club membership. The commitment is a kind of covenant between you and yourself to change your self-image, for the reasons you and only you alone can enumerate. More importantly, the Commitment is a way of them telling you that THIS is what they WILL do, as opposed to what they aspire or plan to do or have said they will do. DARN indeed, but what do they believe they WILL actually do? There is a large gap between what people intend to do, and what they finally commit to do, given the challenge to the underlying image we have of ourselves. Think NYE resolutions. The extent to which these two things relate depends on how well established their sense of purpose has become in relation to what they dream about and what they will in fact strive to achieve toward those dreams. And what you dream of being is often out of sync with your inner view of who you are now.

Goal Setting

You can see from Philippa and Vick's goal setting that things cannot be superficial if you want to drive change, change the way you eat, move, sleep, plan, and bring up your children. Goal setting, according to the literature, is a great way to help make your aspirations come true. Goals are written, personal, progressive, and achievable, have a definite time line, and should include people who can help you get there. The planning of them should fulfil, if the self-determination guys have it right, three criteria: **importance, confidence, and relatedness**.

Importance:

In keeping with the idea of mastery, you have to decide why something is intrinsically motivating for you, something that will galvanize your resolve to change, get you fired up, serves your greater purpose in life, serves your self-image in a positive way. To do that, you must be clear as to why this thing, this goal that you have now formulated, is vitally important, a cherished, cannot-live-without-it goal in keeping with your view of your inner life. Having determined you want to do something, need to do it, you must be clear on the 'why' element: more importantly, the overall 'why' of your life's direction, why the gnawing pain of your self-image is driving this change.

As with Philippa and Vick above, becoming clear on your emotional drivers' importance to you at this stage of your life is the key to adopting it and sticking with the goal to completion.

Let us look at someone else, for instance:

Charles. At sixty was doing well, but ate out often, at a lot of conferences and business dinners and lunches. He found that he had gained about a kilogram of weight each year for a few decades more or less, so he was quite overweight. Diet after diet was started, but he was not able to sustain the weight loss. When I asked him why lose weight? he said the usual things: health, fit in clothes, standard replies like that. One of my therapists drilled down deeper. He began to speak of his son getting married, that a grandchild was on the way, and divorced, he was feeling lonely. Pushing him further, the biggest reason was the need to keep earning money as his investments had crashed a bit with the GFC. He needed to insure his son and grandchild's future, provide for them, find a new girlfriend to share his life with, all of which could now be more clearly linked to his future weight-loss goals, and timelines set to them. It worked. His purpose overwhelmed his hesitations. His self-image emerged, and created a sense of unease about where he now was, and pushed him forward, meaningfully.

It is not enough to set a goal and want or need it: it should be a most cherished, compelling goal, wanting it more than anything in the world, given it will contribute to your greater endeavour in your world and work, and drive a new image of yourself. Charles would ask himself, when in front of the pastry shelf in the coffee shop, "Do I want this cake more than anything else in the world, more than my family security?" He would refer to his cue cards in his wallet, and say to himself, "No, I want other things more, at a level beyond my immediate reality" and he could walk away, taking his now cherished image of himself to safety.

Confidence: the opposite to ambivalence

Allied to mastery, to the getting good at something you treasure, it is important to keep ambivalence under control and not create discrepancy. Ambivalence is created by realizing a life-direction, purposeful big goal might be really quite distant in time, too far in advance to stir your motivation, out of keeping with how you actually view yourself; it may be a large leap that you have failed at before, leaving you wondering at your own ability, lowering your confidence, with the "on the one hand, but on the other" discussion with yourself. Who am I really, you may be asking of the wardrobe image inside: dress me in the colours I most deserve?

Now imagine you are about to go to a college. The course will run three years. You have finished about twelve years of schooling and you have passed. Levels of confidence will be high, since you have passed all twelve prior, why not three or four going forward? No problem your emotions say.

But what if you had failed and repeated two out of the last few years of school? Then your confidence levels would run afoul with a few negative emotions, and you would not be sure that you could get your degree. You would concentrate on each semester, accumulating successes and gaining confidence, or changing or substituting subjects along the way to play to your strengths.

The same applies to effective goal setting. Each goal, as you set it contains within it a set of sub-goals or micro goals, small steps to toward the end goal. Concentrating on these mini-achievements helps support a sense of mastery, a sense of gradually getting better at what you are trying to accomplish in the end, and scaffolding your self-image. You can see the value of staying focussed. Setting out with a sense of purpose will mean you have a touchstone to evaluate each step of each plan you set that has, as its final outcome, a featured desire for your life, a clear image of who you want to be, inside, not to others only, but a connection between you and the others who are watching, or should be.

Set micro goals of three months or less

My colleague Prof Russ Barkley, who is well known for his books on Attention Deficit disorders, has a publication hidden somewhere in his garage (or so he tells me). This work showed that when we think forward in time this is accompanied by increasing activation of the prefrontal cortex in the brain – a wave of activation that moves forward heading for the front of the brain until it stops at the pole: in a healthy thirty something adult this spread of activation would stretch ahead about 11–12 weeks. I will give you the exact study when Prof Russ cleans out his boxes. This could take a while, so read on, okay?

This means that beyond about three months, as you will recall from the desire to cram for mid-term exams in college, nothing stirs our imagination when it comes to fitness goals. This is also the cut-off point beyond which we start to see results in the gym, or from a really healthy diet, and so on.

This means that a goal to lose weight, or get to the gym, or learn a language may be pushing the limits beyond the point where the brain can get continuously more excited. Setting your micro goals, your milestones towards successful adoption of a healthy behaviour, should limit expected time of goal success to three months distant or less, and support the maintenance of your image of who you are growing to be.

So if you know you can lose half a kilogram, or about 1.1lbs of weight per week, and you need to drop twenty-four pounds, then set goals of four pounds per month, and celebrate each four-pound goal success as if it were the end goal. Looking ahead six months to your twenty pounds still to lose goal may not excite you as much as losing four pounds in the next month, and celebrating that, and the six similar events of four pounds each. Small jumps in self-image, not losing sight of who and where you are change-wise along the way.

Each month that goes by reinforces your confidence that what you are doing is making a difference, and you should not ignore these important small milestones; each in themselves an important step.

So when you set your goals, each time a major goal presents, far in time and effort, cut it up into a series of mini-events, each in its own right a step to eventual goal success. Celebrate each small milestone, as if it were the end.

Readiness

Most of us know how a weekend of binge eating and drinking makes us feel by Sunday night: guilty? Monday is 'diet start' day, or so it seems listening to the Sunday night aspirations or the Saturday night bargaining about 'Monday, I will pay for this by dieting' day.

> *When you have approached a goal properly, and established at a deep level exactly why this is emotionally a most cherished and vital event; and once you have worked out the baby steps that will get you there without the lofty goal deflating your motivation, with between where you are now and where you want to go sorted out, and once your self-image can feel what it is like at getting better and better at doing the stuff you see as vital, then you will have the moxie to get off your complacent butt and do it.*

You have to ignite some readiness, some activation ignition. As Mel Robbins notes, you will not feel like it much, but certainly the two steps above will have helped move you somewhat and given you the confidence that it can succeed if you start sometime. The time would be now. In her terms, the five-second rule applies: if you want to do something and hesitate longer than a few seconds, this might leave you stuck where you are now. However, when you have worked the above two criteria well, you will be less stuck.

The point here is, in a year henceforth, will you be happy that:

1. You started now or.

2. You did nothing now?

Well, the answer to that was simple. Would you be happy you waited? Most unlikely.

Starting is everything, so the willingness or readiness to start is vital to the process. Who can help you start NOW, who is most likely to come to your rescue? **You**.

Recall the DARN-C story above? I mentioned that the C was a contract you write down. Here is what it looks like:

Commitment: DARN-Contract

1. Write down the top ten reasons why this goal is the most cherished of all.

2. Rewrite them in rank order, most important to the least important.

3. Choose the top three and write them down under the heading of **Importance.**

4. Now dissect each goal into the micro goals that make it up, and make sure the timeline for each does not exceed eleven to twelve weeks, or break them up further. Write these goals down under the heading **Confidence**.

5. Write down all the reasons you can think of for why you should start now, this very day, and not tomorrow. Rank order them and write the top three down under the heading **Readiness to Change**.

6. If you can think of anyone who can help you accomplish these things, write their names down under a heading **Relatedness**.

Now sign and date it. These are your goals, and you can commit to them, because you can come back to them and change them if you need. This is change on your own terms, no one else's. Most importantly, write down what you think you REALLY will do. If it is not enough, go back and look at the points 1-6 again until you feel you will do it.

Now, what will you actually do?

The issue that still remains is although the DARN is done, the C part to come is about what you will actually now go and really do. The gap as I mentioned between intended and actual is quite significant. Looking at all you have written is fine and good, but what will the outcome actually be? In immersing yourself in a really committed relationship with yourself on significant change, you might need to contemplate further:

NOW: on a scale of one to ten, think of how it will feel if you do not manage your commitment? On the other hand, how good will it feel on a scale of one to ten if you do manage to achieve what you set out to do? Finally, on a scale of one to ten how great will it feel if you exceed your goals in all manner of ways, how will that feel? Write it down, and you have your commitment written more in emotional terms, rather than pure practicality.

You have a series of statements that defines your purpose now, and should fit in with your overall life goal. How important it is to you, how confident you are that you can master the process and achieve what you need to do, and finally, how you will compel yourself to begin immediately, and who can help you achieve this? Supporting your sense of self-efficacy, you will achieve your purpose: A new self-image.

At most points in this process, you will have to balance the positives and negatives to make some decisions. A decisional balance matrix may help you do this. Let us see how to test your commitment to real, meaningful, significant change.

Decisional Balance Matrix for Breaking Ambivalence

Every decision to do something healthy involves an upside, and a downside. Secondly, any decision to do nothing involves the same, an upside and a downside. Draw up a decisional balance matrix of four quadrants in two rows, from the authors of motivational interviewing techniques:

Label the four quadrants this way: fill in the shaded areas:

	Advantages	Disadvantages
Doing Nothing		
Changing Things		

Let's say it looks like this when you are done:

	Advantages	Disadvantages
Doing Nothing	No Effort; Eat what I like; Drink what I like; maintain status quo; relax a lot	Poor health; shorter life; doctor's bills; less income as I age; diabetes, arthritis
Changing Things	Live Longer and happier; more income over years; less disability; more vitality and enjoyment; praise from others	Lots of effort; have to do a lot different; failure threat; need help; will test my willpower

Now you tell yourself:

The block – **Changing Things/Advantage**s – is what you will have if you change things now.

The block – **Doing Nothing/Disadvantages** – is in reality what you will experience if you carry on as you do now.

The block – **Changing Things/Disadvantages** – contains the roadblocks you have to overcome.

The block – **Doing Nothing/Disadvantages** – contains all of your bad habits that must change.

The future is clear, and in accordance with the principal of autonomy, you are the expert in you, so change on your own terms, or leave things the way they are forever: do the above exercise and see how you fare. Again, shining the light on the prism of ambivalence, these four shaded blocks above are the way to shine in the future, and not land up where you do not want to be health or disability-wise.

> *This future is in your hands, and no one is coming to rescue you, but you yourself, and that is a good thing, as you are the expert in you, remember?*

Things to remember:

- When it comes to change, you are the final authority on how well you do, and how best to proceed: trust yourself

- Any expert who says they have the solution is missing a very important point: they are just visiting your life. You are living it, and know best what works for you.

- When you establish a goal, it is natural to feel that this may not work out: break it up into stuff you feel confident you can achieve in the shorter term, and work gradually toward the big scary, off-putting future one.

- The long journey is accomplished, step by baby step, not in big leaps, where you break your legs each time you land.

- Change should be on your own terms, for your own reasons, not anybody else's.

- What you want from people is not a web of inspired speech, but a warm relationship that supports your self-image in changing for the best. That includes your personal trainer or friend or partner in life. They are visiting your life; you are the one who has to live it.

- No one on their death bed says, oh, I should have spent more time at work, or smoking, or sitting around, do they? Do they? Seriously?

- There will often be a gap between what you commit to, and what you finally attempt or succeed in. This is normal, not something to regret.

- Look to define a purpose to your life trajectory. Is the lifestyle you are now leading entirely aligned with this greater purpose? Or is there a negative churning, emotional element that derails you, or threatens to derail you? Let's deal with that threat to your self-image.

Chapter Five

bLUe

building a positive psychology is not the same as being positive

harlie came to see me, dying of cancer. Forced to sell his hardware business, where he had spent twelve hours a day becoming a multimillionaire, he did not know how to spend the last few months available to him: "I have made a living, but never lived." Falling asleep at the wheel on the way home one night, the CT scan on his unconscious head revealed a left frontal tumour. This was cleaned up, but being in the left orbitobasal-frontal area, they could not clear out all of it: it would grow back. Charlie had a wife and grown children he hardly knew, and now could barely produce speech. He had $16million in the bank and was dying, almost without a voice, with no image left of who or what he had been, or would become. After some motivational interviewing, and a six-week body-brain program, Charlie decided to rebuild his ageing, now damaged and neglected 1984 Porsche 911 so he could finally part with it on good terms before he died. Lying on the floor of his 'workshop' *(do not get me wrong, it had a marble floor, a Ducati on a platform, and the Porsche had a special ramp!) night and day, he managed to restore the car to concourse pristine condition in four months. Selling it for an astounding 200% of what he paid new, he found himself with nothing to do, after getting his legal-financial affairs in order. His son told him of another bashed up Porsche Turbo in a nearby panel beater's yard, so he bought that, and started over, this time with his mechanic son's assistance. His wife commented, a year to the day after he was supposed to not live much longer: "I have never seen Charlie so motivated, happy, funny, and filled with vitality". A review of his tumour shows it is growing very slowly, and another operation might be needed in a year or two, but the doctors are pretty happy with him. Charlie's first language was not English, and he struggles to speak English now, preferring his mother tongue: German. His previously estranged wife and children have learned some more of this, helping him communicate further. Charlie acknowledges that of all the training he received from me, the Positive Psychology interventions were the key. "When I had to work out what I was grateful for, what three good things I had done that day, it was always around family and Ferdinand Porsche... not necessarily in that order!" The German sense of humour.*

The Science of Positivity

Positivity is not some hippie view of life, about some positive affirmation, such as: "I am happy, healthy, and I feel terrific". These would not have helped Charlie survive or reverse the inflammatory cytokines and interleukins that changed his gene expression to cancer, recurring bouts of drinking and depression, adultery, things which had ruined his father's life, ending in his father's suicide when the Russians closed in on Berlin. His father, a *Waffen SS* officer, had died before Charlie knew him.

In the face of dire threat or past failures, facing a mirror and saying wonderful things about you to yourself does not do much at all when you have to confront your inner view of your self-image. Positive psychology is not about slogans or bumper stickers or writing *Go For It* on your cleats. These do help, but do not fundamentally change the inner view of you when you critique yourself and your history to date.

Positive Psychology developed largely out of Marty Seligman growing weary of the constant flow of misery that entered his consulting rooms day after day. Like reading entrails, many psychologists find themselves wary of trafficking in human misery, while physically disintegrating by sitting hour after hour listening to negative people wading in their own sadness and loss. Worse, therapy stutters along when that happens.

Whilst psychologists such as I will acknowledge how rewarding it is to see people emerge, grow, pay their bill, hug us goodbye and move on, it is a weighty profession. With a misleading portrayal in the popular media notwithstanding, psychologists have the same problems as others in their daily lives, and as my friend David Manchester says, therapy is a young man's game, it is so taxing.

Enter the Positive Psychologists. Seligman, Frederickson, Mihaly Csikszentmihalyi and others, who began to study whether the science of misery was trumped by the science of positivity. In many ways, it was. Not just depressive patients: Seligman has been given hundreds of millions of dollars to bring this science to the US military.

Let us examine one of his interventions. You think of a person who you knew before, and who has made a major contribution to your life. You never thanked them. So now you write a three hundred word thank-you letter to them explaining what they did at that time. Then you track them down, and force them to listen to you read your thank-you note. Patients who did this were less depressed. Facebook makes this a simple and public task.

Here is another. You come to the end of your day. You lie in bed with your journal, and write down three great things that happened to you that day. Then you elaborate on the things you did that day, which led to those three good occurring outcomes. Later you write how you will continue to make this happen the next day. Patients who did this were less depressed.

Let us go back to a sense of self-efficacy. On a daily basis, we are confronted with images of worldly events we have NO control over: climate, politics, distant wars, looming financial catastrophes, and so on. They elicit non-conscious negative responses from us, over which we have no control, but, which become the filters through which we interpret modern life events, a selective negative bias. Looking at life through lenses that filter out light.

The positive psychologists worked out using mathematical models that for each such negative input, as in events we cannot control, we need three equally positive inputs to counter them. However, should this be in the context of a relationship, such as a marriage, we would need a 5:1 positive to negative input ratio; in a group, such as a workplace or sports team, we would need 11:1 events to support a reasonably positive self-image, when things get tough.

Are we are hardwired to be miserable? Yes, and it makes us sick!

In terms of how we developed across time, there is not much advantage to organisms being overwhelmingly positive. Lying basking in the sun without a care in the world does not help you prepare for the ice age: being nervous and neurotic, learning how to make fur clothes and start fires does help when the 'you-know-what' hits the fan. Negativity does not drive change. Mlle Laurent must know that smoking French women are dying like flies, but it does not motivate her to change, but has the opposite effect as her smoking is rewarded, or, she shrugs her shoulders and tries to avoid getting hit by a Citroen while crossing the road, or other hazards.

Hardwired into our perception of the world, non-conscious perceptions occur within a few hundred milliseconds, long before we become consciously aware, at about 300–500 milliseconds, that something has happened. By the time we are aware, let us say that a cute blonde girl has walked into our peripheral vision, our brain has already processed that vision and alerted us to the value of that vision before us. By the time we realise that the girl is young enough to be our daughter, and regards us as some creepy old guy who is eeeeeuuuuwww, our bodies have responded with some sense of desire. The lower elements of the brain do not know what an inappropriate response is: they simply alert us to events in our environment, and the breeding potential of a young woman is a very salient event. Hence producers will have responded to Mlle Laurent's beauty and animated voice and face before her smoking habit. They are looking for an actress, not a smoking advert.

So the amygdala and other emotional regulating centres are quick to react with fear and disgust, with a very powerful physical-physiological response, which occurs a few hundred milliseconds before we can think effectively about something.

Happiness and content are low arousal emotions and as such are not likely to save our lives. Focusing on hunting a deer or gazelle in the savannah to the exclusion of all else will get you killed by a predator. Sleeping deeply and not being jumpy and hypervigilant will get you killed, if not in the savannah, then certainly on an LA Freeway. Small dogs are jumpy and yappy, big ones less so, and so they sleep more deeply. Our deep emotional processing systems are akin to very small, reptilian, jumpy, yapping dogs.

The hormones of being alert and ready to freeze, run away, or fight and bleed are adrenalin and cortisol. These are not health-inducing hormones, but they have a strong effect on us physically to keep us in fight, flight or freeze mode in the short term.

The nervous system and negativity vs. positivity

The part of the nervous system that supports these activities is the sympathetic branch of the Autonomic Nervous System (ANS). The other parts are the parasympathetic and the enteric.

The sympathetic tone of the system, maintained with accompanying alertness in the Beta wave electrical activity of the brain, is one of arousal. The heart beat is regular, each beat peak on the EEG records pretty much the same distance from the last, and from the next. In those who are trained as Special Forces soldiers, this is accompanied with high levels of Neuropeptide Y, and they cope beautifully with the stress of combat. However, they die young. This arousal, this metronomic heartbeat, does not guarantee a long life. Cautiously scared people live longer in combat, but over time, both Special Forces operatives and the highly anxious and depressed die younger than they should.

On the other hand, parasympathetic dominance, that of rest and digest, is healthy, and indicative of low arousal, of Alpha activity in the brain, of a calm and irregular heartbeat: yes, the beat to beat measure is different between one beat and the next. This sinus arrhythmia is healthier than the metronomic heartbeat. And it can be induced by breathing a certain way, knows as Respiratory Sinus Arrhythmia... more of that later.

So stress is not healthy in modern life terms, as chronic stressors, exacerbated at times by moving house, divorce, death of a loved one, financial woes, all attack our health as they overwhelm some pre-set setpoint beyond which our physiology deforms and we get ill.

These are inflammatory conditions at the cellular level. It is accepted that many mental conditions such as depression are inflammatory conditions, and in turn, depression and other mood and anxiety conditions are independent risk factors for mortality, such as heart disease. Negativity and unhappiness are fatal in the long run. Feeling overwhelmed is the equivalent of 5 cigarettes a day in health risk.

Negativity:

A non-conscious negative bias predicts a large range of unhealthy body and brain behaviours. This means that the first few milliseconds of automatic self-defending responses are not healthy. Hence, as Beck and later cognitive therapists described, addressing this negativity is a key to both mental and more bodily health. As you are aware by now, these entities are one and the same.

Let us see how we are hardwired.

By the time we have realised we have seen something, or heard it, our brains have been busy. In the first few hundred milliseconds, our brain is assessing what we see or hear, whilst working out if it is dangerous, or of significance or not. This is called emotional valence, or salience.

If what we see is dangerous, e.g. a speeding car or a sabre tooth tiger, we are galvanized to move quickly out of the way. We are in reality, priming our muscles to get going fractions of a second before we know what it is. Think of ducking down out of the way of a flying ball or swooping bird almost without you realizing it.

But by 500 milliseconds, you are, in fact, processing that information more consciously. However, if your brain has already determined that this information was somehow threatening, your conscious thoughts will have to work with this negatively valanced or flagged material.

We all have this system, which screens and evaluates information for threat, namely in an attempt to minimize surprising danger, and maximise final outcomes in our favour. On the other hand, if this information is overwhelming valued as positive, subsequent negative ideation might not turn us away from the attraction, or it might, if we tend to be disposed to negativity, finding something wrong in every silver lining. If change supports our self-image, it will move us along well enough.

There is a lot of information coming in every second, some positive, some negative in relation to that vital image we have of our self, that self-attribution factor I mentioned before.

Should however your brain be hardwired for **singling out** information from the environment that is negatively valanced, that you assess as likely to provide a threat of some kind, then this is termed a negativity bias. Positive events are neglected or interpreted as negative. Given the blindness of the system, it may find a tremendous amount falsely threatening. As Montaigne noted, he had lived through many disasters, both big and small, most of which... never happened at all. Most of what we worry about actually never happens, but we allocate a lot of resource to worry as a type of problem solving strategy, albeit not a great way to do that.

Your brain therefore will constantly have to consciously deal with incoming information that is selectively biased by an early and lightning-fast non-conscious evaluation system. Overwhelmingly, your interpretations of the world will be that it is a nasty place.

Not surprisingly, Aaron Beck and his followers found that a substantial amount of brain-based pathology included a tendency to be negatively biased. This was not helpful caution, but a tendency to interpret the majority of events in daily life in some negative way.

Angela was livid. In a lowly paid job well below her station in life, she discovered fortnightly money coming into her account with no indication as to where it was from. Berating her bank manager, she finally found out that she had been awarded an increase in her pay packet retrospectively, and this was adjustment coming through as back-pay. "Why did they not tell me these things! I spent hours on the phone!" Sigh.

Instead of being happy with her increase, Angela found it irritating, as she did with most things. When her cousin Dot failed to show for a coffee meeting one morning, Angela bit her nails to a shred believing something horrible must have happened, rather than Dot's car failing to start and her mobile phone battery being flat. The idea that Dot hated her suddenly was more in keeping with her overall negative world and self-image interpretations.

For Angela and others with high levels of negativity bias, the worst interpretation of daily events dominates their automatic 'stinking thinking' as some experts call it. Closely related to the older concept of neuroticism, negativity has its roots in personality style and anxiety. More troubling, it has been implicated as predicting all kinds of ill health and disability.

The therapy termed Cognitive Behaviour Therapy was developed to deal with such negatively biased interpretations of the world, given the high levels of anxiety and mood disorders as well as physical illness in people so predisposed. This would include early life events perceived as stressful, which could even predispose someone to Post Traumatic Stress Disorder later in life for instance.

Negativity is also surprisingly contagious. When my Professor walked into his unit where I worked, he would know immediately if a patient with high levels of negative bias had been admitted. When his favourite nurses snapped at him, the psychologist went home with a headache, and the ward clerk began to overeat, he would know: "Ann is here, he used to grumble... I would bet on it". Ann was our local professional patient who regularly checked in for booster shots, and rapidly made everyone miserable, especially when she had a new love of her life, who she was convinced would dump her any time soon.

Infectious negativity in a workplace is termed presenteeism. Such workers – and recall more than 80% of people who are depressed are not only at work, but engaged in being happily negative – make those around them work harder. They have to face the negativity from others and within themselves, and fight to re-interpret a lot of what they are getting from the moody person. Since I noted above one needs 11:1 good to bad things in ratio terms, imagine how pervasive negative interpretations are in the workplace, and how hard they are to counteract, when a miserable person comes to work every day, sharing this negativity.

Parents looking to protect children by pointing out the downside to absolutely everything are also promoting anxiety and negativity, not a careful and successful exploration of the options available to us: worry is not an effective way to become an assertive and positive solver of tricky challenges and protect children from error. As Einstein noted, the thinking styles of today will not help us deal with the challenges of tomorrow, or the solutions of the 20th Century. Remember, this was said in the last century.

Overcoming a negative bias

This takes some doing but it is worth it.

Gratitude

This is not just a counting of the blessings, but a serious attempt to retrain the brain into automatic positivity. Instead of the negative filtering of information, the preference being given to finding the negative out there and shovelling it to the forefront, gratitude trains the brain to find the positive and put it into the forefront, and also make a habit of doing that.

Something my patients loved doing were gratitude rituals based on finding special things in their lives and writing them down, focusing on them often.

However, I found many people could not find a positive event anywhere. Some people really have difficult lives!

For this group, I developed this mundane ritual. This means taking three minutes each day when they woke up to look at the most common objects around them, and determine why life without them would be nasty. Later, they find this makes them more successful in looking for events and explanations that will drive them onward and upward to better things.

Ann arrived at work the night after Kevin dumped her, ending a three-year engagement to be married. Prone to negativity, she had learned the mundane ritual some years before, during an episode of depression. As she sat at her desk, it kicked in. "My stapler – life without you would be papers getting muddled and costing me hours. My Toyota – do you recall the cost of my Mercedes services?! And those warm cloth seats compared to those cold hard leather ones? And as for the trunk, love the roomier one I have now. My Chapstick – I simply could not live with dry lips for more than two minutes. My tea – need I say more, the taste, the comfort". Despite the tragedy of loss she felt, two days of resorting to this silliness, which her brain was trained to do for just about everything 24/7, every time she thought of him, and her loss, helped her escape out of the moment.

Paul was injured playing his best game for years, and soon learned that he could never play again. He began to drink, slumped around, stayed up all night and slept during the day. Finally, he arrived in therapy (he had been before years ago) and said I had better fix him, and he only had one session left in him. He agreed to do whatever I said, so I used one of Martin Seligman's interventions: the letter.

The client is instructed to go home and write a 300 word letter of gratitude to someone from the past, someone who influenced their lives tremendously, and whom they never acknowledged or thanked.

For Paul, it was his first coach. He wrote and revised the letter for a day or two, and then had to follow the rest of the ritual. Tracking down the coach, he convinced him that he would fly to the state he lived in, and would come to visit him 'for a good reason'. The coach was bewildered, now in his late eighties, but he finally agreed. Paul read the letter carefully aloud, while the old man wept. Paul wept too. They spoke of his injury, of his childhood, of the coach's belief that Paul had not learned a damn thing from him. They parted, soaked in nostalgia, and Paul flew home. Paul noted that his misery left him at the coach's door. It was such a great thing to do for his old coach. Paul decided to carry on using his fame for good, turning to society to find ways to leave the world a better place.

Doing things for other people is a powerful incentive. Just watching a video of Mother Theresa helping others is enough to boost your metabolism intensely resulting in an enhanced immune system, or so the research goes.

Smiling at three strangers a day may seem weird for those in modern commuting circles, but it works nicely. Just doing three random nice things for three random strangers a day is valuable too. It establishes your self-image as one who gives without taking.

Why? We are gregarious creatures, but more importantly, we developed the capacity to be highly affected by the moods and feelings of others. I will take this up later.

Smiling and Humour

You may have noticed that telling a joke that you borrowed off a stand-up comedian may fall flat when you try it. It was funny at the time, but not later on. Or you did not tell it right, you think?

Actually, we are more likely to laugh at a joke or funny sitcom if we are in the company of a crowd of others, than if alone or with only one another. A room full of laughing people has a life of its own.

In the one-to-one setting, people who tell jokes all the time are just annoying, as they push us away from a close relationship or access to their emotions that way. The life and soul of the party who is never serious is not a great person to have a close and meaningful relationship with.

Speakers telling a joke are more likely to laugh at it than the audience. In an audience, you are thirty times more likely to laugh at a joke than if you are on your own. Even chimpanzees laugh, and can laugh while breathing in as well as breathing out, a form of panting, which we cannot do. Humour is crafted in our genes as a form of instinctive social bonding. And speaking of which, you cannot tickle yourself either. That takes someone else to do for you.

Victims of stroke with facial paralysis cannot smile, but when tickled or told a joke, usually a smile or laughter occurs as before; laughter is generated in the brainstem as with other essential functions and may suppress stress hormones and elevate antibodies. It encourages us to play well with each other – tickling a baby, for instance, lays the foundation for a behaviour that carries over into the social life of the baby as an adult. The surprise touch of an adult on a baby or child becomes the surprise of a punch line later as adults face a comedian. Stimulating the nucleus accumbens, an ancient dopamine-based pleasure centre in the brain triggers laughter, an addictive centre. We are not reacting to punch lines in responding to a joke, but to the sense of social connectedness it brings. Such a playful thing as tickling is only typical of mammals, higher animals.

Another thing about laughter: it is an honest social signal that is hard to fake and babies can laugh by the age of four months. It can also be used cruelly to reinforce a group's solidarity by mocking deviants and insulting outsiders; people in a one-down situation socially are more likely to laugh at jokes, especially when the teller of the joke is a superior, the boss. Laugher helps with blood pressure, heart rate, breathing, catecholamines, cortisol, and growth hormone regulation.

A British research group set out to find the funniest joke of life. It was decided finally that the best one occurred during a recording of a *Goon Show* for the BBC:

911 Operator: What is your emergency?

Caller: A man has been shot!

911 Operator: Is he breathing?

Caller: I am not sure.

911 Operator: Is he dead?

Caller: I am not sure.

911 Operator: Can you make sure for me?

Caller: Hold on... *sound of footsteps fading away, then a gunshot... then footsteps returning.*

Caller: He is now!

Another researcher put his depressed patients in front of a TV for a whole weekend, and only showed them the full season of Seinfeld episodes. It worked, compared to medication, to reduce depression quite significantly and quickly.

However, it is not just guffawing in front of a TV or comic that is healthy.

Smiling does it too: however, we must compare smiling falsely as a sales clerk might, to real smiling, as your grandmother might.

Smiling of the Pan American Airlines type, called the 'Pan Am' smile, is the false smile of the diva welcoming you to her party, or of the cabin crew inviting you on board a fourteen-hour flight, or the family welcoming you, the child welfare inspector, into their home.

Critical to the healthy smile is the *Duchenne* type of smile. This involves a genuine crinkling around the eye, specifically the muscles of *zygomaticus major* and *orbicularis oculi* in the upper face and around the eye. When subjects were given the same picture of a man portraying either the Pan Am or *Duchenne* smiles, they showed overwhelmingly they would favour and trust the man with the real smile. When others smile, we look instinctively to the eyes and the crow's feet, and if there are none, we act as if our lives depended on it in the past, and it probably did: we do not trust or like them.

So smiling sincerely is vital to engaging with others, and that is healthy, as I note later in a chapter dedicated to connections with others.

More vitally, smiling is connected with mood and sudden death.

Barbara Frederickson is a veteran of the Positive Psychology movement, and its extensive research base. One of the more startling findings in those who survived heart attacks was the danger of not smiling genuinely. In those patients who seldom smiled or who smiled typically in an insincere fashion, she notes you can virtually see the heart muscle dying.

Marsha Linehan and her colleagues work extensively with Borderline Personality Disorder, a very challenging set of neurological, childhood issues, and mood and personality conditions rolled up into one in a patient, making it difficult to treat them. However, the challenging half smile, somewhere between a grin and not smiling at all, just using the *zygomaticus* and *orbicularis* to lift the corners of the mouth is enough to lift mood, as her trainers went on to teach me in their workshops.

Try being miserable about something, then go to the mirror and practice the twitchy half smile, just lifting the corners of the lips upward. It is very hard to carry on being miserable.

Jonno was a great rugby football player who peaked young. Depression and drug abuse accompanied his early success, as he left his family and friends behind to play in the big city. Nine years later, broke, injured, using 900mg of a major antipsychotic drug to sleep and with a diagnosis of Bipolar Disorder, he volunteered to be on the TV show I co-hosted. Behind the scenes I taught this 6'4"man to stand up straight and tall, and use assertive language to feed back to his brain and learn optimism in Seligman's terms. After all, I told him, if you young men are not in the front line when danger comes, what will people like me do? But importantly, he learned to look up into the mirror and half smile: it elevated his mood by ten per cent each morning.

The Three Good Things Ritual

Apart from the gratitude, there are many negative inputs coming each day to support a negative bias developing. So often, we are subjected to management, clients, coaches, and other forces out there, which are hell-bent on changing us to work better for them, rather than ourselves, pointing out our inevitable connection to things that go wrong.

This ritual of the positive psychologists is designed to connect us to the good things that we do, and take some ownership of them, by adjusting our own self-image.

It involves sitting quietly with our journal at the end of the day and thinking back on the day's events to single out three awesome things that happened.

We write them down. Then we have to work out what it was that we did to make them happen. What actions did we take to make them come about? What was our role in each of these three amazing events? What proactive learned behaviour made us go out and drive these things to happen? This places our self-image in a decent context.

Then we have to work out how we will get more of the same or similar happening the next day, and the next.

At the end of each week we have twenty more groovy events to reflect on, and more so, to reflect on how we made them come to be. Each day we will learn what skills we have that create good connections to good things, and thus our role in a better, more positive world. Yes, others will point out where we were connected to errors and events, but that is their job not ours. Beating up on ourselves is not our job: so give it up. The end of the day is ours to indulge in being awesome.

So being positive is not exactly useful in keeping us alert and aware of danger, but the world is so full of bad things that we absorb, like the evening news, that we have to do some recovery and regeneration work to overcome the forces against happiness and positivity.

Seligman is now calling it 'Flourishing'. This is more than being passively happy; it is a way of growing yourself beyond the clutches of daily existence.

Flourishing builds resilience and is also protective of your health

Seligman describes various aspects of self-image and health secondary to a Positive Psychology approach:

- Positive people take positive action and lead healthier lifestyles, take better care of themselves, and follow good advice.

- Positive people attract strong friendships and family support, and lonely people are markedly less healthy.

- The immune system produces more T-lymphocytes and other indicators of health in positive people.

Finally: a longitudinal study of the intensity of smiling on the 1952 Baseball Register photograph demonstrated that the more genuine and intense smiles predicted accurately how long each smiler would live. The rot starts early and so smiling and genuinely investing in others in a happy and positive way builds the seeds of a longer and healthier life. Think how bad anger and negativity must be in the opposite way – not a good way to live your shorter life.

Now happier people smile more, and those that smile live longer. Those who seek happiness, live longer. Those who expect happiness and expect to live longer, do.

You might say, well my life isn't happy. Here is a story for you.

Jewish wisdom says that a man approaches his creator and asks how he might recognize a happy man, and how to find him in the first place. Look for the happy man he is told, and borrow his shirt and then you will know why he is happy. So the man sets out and finally sees a bare chested man ploughing his fields, singing away, clearly happy. He tries to borrow his shirt, but finds the man is too poor to own one.

Poor people are often found to be more satisfied with life than others would expect. When you come to the end of the day, living hand to mouth, and at the end of each day you have a roof over your head and your family is fed, you tend to be genuinely content, more so than a billionaire driving home in his Aston Martin, who cannot quite put his finger on what he has accomplished that day. Over the years, my therapy room has been filled with beautiful and rich people who simply wanted to die. A study has shown that two years after winning the Lotto or landing in a wheelchair, both groups are equally content with their lives. That is a great example of intrinsic motivators and inner worth triumphing over extrinsic superficiality. The hippies had a point. So does Dan Gilbert.

As Dan Gilbert has pointed out, happiness is synthetic.

Making Happiness Happen

If positivity and happiness are not guaranteed in any country's constitution, then we have to go out there and make it happen, synthesize it. We know modern value systems equate early financial success and large houses and fancy cars as the sources of happiness, as well as a constant stream of adoring partners, or fame, or being onstage as a rock star or hero, but sadly most of us will never manage that in our lifetimes, so are we doomed to be miserable?

Take people such as those selected out by Gilbert. Most kids would love to become a pop idol, recognized with hysterical rejoicing such as experienced by The Beatles then, or Justin Bieber now. But what of those who came really close, and lost it?

Pete Best was an original Beatle, dumped by his manager, just as they became the phenomenon they were. Best lost out as a drummer to Ringo Starr. However, he was interviewed many times as you would expect, and affirmed that after his initial shock and misery he went on to a successful music career and achieved great contentment, stating that without doubt he was the happiest of all The Beatles, their success notwithstanding. Of course, by then John and George were dead, Paul had lost a wife to cancer and one to a costly, messy divorce, and is now married for the third time. Ringo has never really shone massively since in the world's eye, but perhaps is as happy as Pete.

Six other quarterbacks were drafted before Tom Brady in the USA, who made it into a team last of all, but his career has since then vastly eclipsed the others, despite the sense of despair he felt initially at being picked after 198 others that year, which still makes him tear up with the recalled pain. He went out for the first year at the Patriots grateful that he was there, even if he did not start for them. However, when he did get on the field, the quarterback he replaced never made it back into the starting line-up. It was Brady who made history, the others, not so much. Brady was able to come back from the worst of times, more than once. Injured in 2008 so badly he did not play, in 2009 during his first return game he threw 378 yards. When they were losing the game, almost at the last moment, he threw two goals quickly and so they won the game, to earn him the title (again and again) of the Comeback Kid of all time. Having lost the Superbowl this year in 2012, and hanging his head in despair, it is clear that despite his successes, more than just about anyone else in history apart from Joe Montana, his goals are still vital and cherished for him, and are still emotive drivers of his success, with no complacency.

You will recall this chapter started out with Charlie and his Porches? He had to remake his life in a manner that he never dreamed of until his life was threatened, and now makes the most of his world, loving each day. He understands that he has to work on his happiness, which did not come naturally or spontaneously for most of his life until the scourge of brain cancer emerged after a traumatic brain event that knocked him unconscious. This was the best thing that ever happened to him.

For Charlie and others, they will use the phrase "I guess it all turned out for the best" not because they sat and waited for the tide to turn, but because they stopped, dropped, and rolled when things caught fire. Literally, they looked around and took action. When you do that, something else happens, as it does when Charlie works on his cars:

"When I am totally busy Doc, consumed, the world just passes me by in a blaze of glory. I realise that hours have passed, and I could not tell you exactly what I did. I see a complete engine block, and have to think hard about how it just magically assembled itself!"

Such a description of the passage of time without effort is common from peak performers, like world-class athletes. They simply go off into another world, so engaged and focused that the world outside of that focus dwindles away to nothing.

Thinking too much for any athlete, especially a baseball batter or pitcher is a barrier to their success. Tom Brady cannot afford to think too much now, any more than can Tiger Woods, if greatness is to be preserved across time. When your resources are gainfully consumed by the demands of the task you have chosen, a task that fulfils your purpose in life, then you experience flow. Yogi Berra said that he could hit, and he could think, but not at the same time.

Flow

My colleague Damian Vaughn works with one of the great positive forces in world psychology, Mihaly Csikszentmihalyi. He says that Flow is the state of total absorption that comes about when skills and challenge are optimally balanced, the experience of working at full capacity, absorbing all of our conscious capability. Clearly, you can see that the presence of negative thought or emotions will disrupt this, and distract from the moment. The moment, and attention to the moment, is part of mindfulness, related to flow. Combining the current moment and linking it to tomorrow's moment, is positive psychology.

A famous set of experiments relate to a man named Walter Mischel at Stanford. Essentially, he tested children by placing an enticing incentive of candy in front of them. He then advised them that delaying their desire to eat the candy would result in a future reward of more candy. Children who delayed the gratification of scooping up the treat not only scored a bigger hit of candy, but when followed up went on to do better than others in real life, demonstrating an ability to avoid a 'prepotent' response in the environment for a more abstract goal that is an ingredient of success for all of us. The sacrifice of the now, or time we spend now, that has a future payoff, a distant, cherished payoff toward which we have to engage all of our energy, is one of the keys to positive lasting change.

Living a positive life is not quite the same as the Protestant work ethic, where hard work in this life is rewarded in some proposed life hereafter. It is about avoiding the demands of the immediate environment (prepotent response) and seeking out a more advantageous future by acting (or not acting) immediately to improve your circumstances beyond the temporal horizon. This is the function of the prefrontal cortex and other executive areas of the brain. As noted in the Motivation section above, we can all think ahead and simulate the future, choosing behaviours now that will have the best outcome for us in the future: the better and more frequently we do this, the greater our chances of success. Responding to the prepotent moment can be costly, and impulsive.

Being distracted by temporary setbacks, or about what might still come, derails flow and neglects the search for happiness. Negativity has only a protective effect, but slows or derails advance. Flow is as much a position one takes, as much as it is a process of balancing what we believe we can do, with what we perceive must do. You can see the 'believe' and the 'perceive', both not based on facts, but on our perceptions. Perceptions of our self-image, perceptions which believe we have capacity, and perceive the challenge is within the limits of that capacity, create a sense of self-efficacy and reduce stress. Believing the worst is coming is anxiety, believing the worst has already happened is depression. Being mindful of the task at hand is Flow, a form of focus, rather than thought: total engagement.

The balance of belief and perceive is understood as trust, trust in a stable self-image that can cope. When we trust in ourselves and what we can do, irrespective of past evidence or future fears, outcomes are possible which deny the past and affirm the future. Again, it is scaffolding your self-image that counts.

It is not about believing in yourself: it is about trusting yourself and your clear self-image of who you are. This means binding positive events across time, using your executive functions over time, choosing and rejecting options as you go, absorbed in the process. Then you score goals!

A major study out of the prestigious Karolinska Institute showed that soccer players who had better executive functions certainly were more likely to score goals or assist in others scoring goals. In sport, we know that athletes have to engage in Flow, getting lost in the things they are doing, and that thinking too much is also an impediment to success. The executive functions are thus a superfast choice mechanism, simulating outcomes, so we can choose the immediate and best responses that have the best outcomes in future seconds. This superfast processing has to operate off a superior non-conscious bias, a self-image which recognises both threat and opportunity quickly, and responds immediately with the best possible choice of action. All of this can be measured using instruments such as CNS Vital Signs, an online neuropsychological assessment battery.

You might think athletes are not the brightest bunch, but it turns out that amongst the peak athletes, the best are also the brightest with the best executive and non-conscious emotional biases which define their self-image as resilient. What makes the best shine is what they do in the most competitive moments, not only against opposing teams, but against their competition for a slot in their own teams. The more competition in a fight to the top, the more we are pushed to excel. When others are fighting with us for scarce resource, that is precisely when trusting ourselves to deliver if we just engage with the best brain we can put forward, directing the best body we can deliver to the contest, pays off. Maintaining a healthy self-image, a realistic but positive appraisal of what we are facing, and what we have to face it with, pays off. This is trust.

So what is this link between a better brain and a better outcome, how do Flow and other concepts fit in?

Firstly, non-conscious emotional bias and simulating outcomes: viz. – thinking, are prone to collide as I have mentioned before, creating ambivalence, where belief and perception are out of synch, leading to a shaky self-image. Thinking says: I want this. Emotions say: it's too hard to accomplish. This is where sportsmen at the peak level excel, in trusting both their capacity and the solubility of the challenge they might face if they just stay true to their skills. This is also why successful people marry the hottest girls.

The thinking part of us includes the motoric, executive functions. These are the bits that can simulate the outcomes of things we can do now, and see which are the most beneficial.

However, in depressed patients we see a lot of failure in that particular skill. One reason, as with athletes, is that thinking is motor, and responds to the non-conscious, bodily emotions with feeling, namely a feeling of those emotions happening, and this disrupts motor activity such as executive functions, so simulating outcomes looks bleak; the war cry of the depressed patient is "There is no future". You can virtually see the failure of the cortical, serotonergic areas to light up. For the anxious, the future looks full of impending danger, driven by dopamine in the lower limbic circuitry.

ADHD kids also seem to have problems with delaying a response, simulating the best outcome, choosing wisely and avoiding the proponent response. When you are incapable of imagining a better future based on what is in front of you, when you cannot simulate in your minds' eye what a good outcome looks like, when it all appears beyond comprehension, then Positivity is impossible, the future is dark, or anxiety provoking.

When the brain appreciates a great deal of sacrifice must be made, and the emotions only provide a bleak picture of what is to come, or what might come, then executive functions fail and all is gloom and doom.

Some people who suffer from an advanced case of negativity will look to a successful outcome and think, "Yeah, like that is ever gonna happen!" making working toward a good outcome most unlikely in simulation terms, and certainly in reality. Being a complete loser or complete failure, looking back and only seeing a succession of failures and projecting that into all future scenarios is not only a failure of self-efficacy, but also of anhedonism: being unable to enjoy anything, part of a depressive presentation.

So in closing, this is why practising positivity skills is not trivial in the face of negativity and the need to minimise our adversity to change, to the threat of meaningful change, and embracing change instead as a way to live a Positive life and maximise opportunity. Bringing the frontal poles of the brain to life is a critical component of the approach.

We are all hardwired to blink when faced with change, to prevaricate. Those who live life in a Positive sense, namely training and building positivity as a source of resilience, will do better both mentally and as I pointed out, physically.

On the other hand, talent shows on TV are full of kids who swagger on stage and say, "My mother told me I can be ANYTHING I want to be" and stomp off stage miffed when the judges kindly point out they should stay at school rather than destroy music any further. They vow to soldier on. We cannot be anything we want to be. You need talent to start and if you want to compete with the best in the world, plenty of that. Secondly, you need to work like a dog, sometimes for ever and ever. Thirdly, timing is everything, and you need to be waiting for luck to come your way by preparing for it. Finally, you have to be selling what people want. Selling positivity is a great way to live. On your death bed, will you say, wow, I should have been more negative, eaten more sometimes food, spent less time with family, I should have been more miserable? I doubt it. Above all else, Positivity as a philosophy seeks ways to do things better, to Flourish in Seligman's words. It is an assertive approach to finding the good stuff, and burning it as fuel.

Joy, Gratitude and Love are some of the elements of Positivity. You can test Positivity by logging onto **http://www.positivityratio.com/single. php** or complete some other similar questionnaires here at **Google: University of Pennsylvania Authentic Happiness Questionnaires.**

Read Seligman's work and that of Barbara Frederickson as well. Chapter eleven of her book sets out a new toolkit developed by herself and others arising from deeper self-study, one's own Eureka moments.

1. ***Tool number one*** in the box is thus to be open to things, as she reiterates again and again. This means really being accepting of what is happening, or what you are thinking, being both aware and accepting of things, looking more at sensory experiences than inner thoughts for instance. Cultivating curiosity and acceptance of current experience without trying or wishing for change, is what

emerges as a goal. Openness thus implies acceptance, experimenting with openness.

2. ***Tool 2*** involves high-quality connections with others. These are life-giving patterns of interaction with others, and recharge in a real physiological change (e.g. Dutton's work), as a result of respectful engagement, helping others succeed, trusting others, and play. Your self-image is interested in the levels of those around you, and defined often in keeping with them.

3. ***Tool 3***: cultivating kindness, five acts of kindness each day, which may be costly, but worthwhile and creative.

4. ***Tool 4***: develop distractions, breaking the grip of a downward pull of rumination and getting away from obsessing over problems, with both healthy and unhealthy distractions possible, avoiding alcohol, junk food, and other unhealthy distractions. Fantasy is not planning, it is just wishing.

5. ***Tool 5***: dispute negative thinking; rooted in cognitive behavioural therapy, with index cards recording the most common negative thoughts we revert to, the voice of ill will. Shuffle the cards, pick one at random, and then rapidly dispute it: what are the facts? Shut down menacing negativity. Work through the deck and become a seasoned disputer of negative thoughts.

6. ***Tool 6***: find nearby nature: good weather should propel us to green or blue, trees, water or sky, which boosts positivity and associates your own image as being part of a greater, global system which has inherent wisdom over the ages.

7. ***Tool 7***: learn and apply strengths, taking Seligman's survey, 240 items, which measures twenty-four character strengths, and how they characterize us in the top five, from **www.authentichappiness.com**. Self-reflection is critical, and the top five given by the toolkit are valuable starters to identify the strengths in a reflective self-portrait.

8. ***Tool 8***: meditate mindfully, daily, for about twenty-five minutes as described in this section.

9. ***Tool 9***: meditate on loving kindness, as described here as well. This is a form of guided, emotional focus, rather than imagery. Reflect on a loved person or pet, arousing warm and tender feelings, and by letting go of the image, and holding the feeling, and extending this inward towards the self, a large hurdle for Westerners. Then it is radiated to others, close, and then wider, to all people and creatures of the earth, globally.

10. ***Tool 10***: ritualize gratitude, by noticing the gifts around us. Describe why each good thing happened, namely the precursors of wonderful events.

11. ***Tool 11***: savour positivity, needing a source of genuine love, pride, etc., and secondly, a willingness to think differently about it now, and then enriching that moment by stretching and amplifying them, tuning oneself to expect good events in advance.

12. ***Tool 12***: visualize your future; imagining yourself ten years from now, imaging what has turned out good, if all current dreams came true, achieving one's best

possible outcomes, and describing this in detail. Draw out the drivers for life, the meaning of existence, all in a journal, accepting deepest hopes and dreams, providing a mission statement, and putting it to a Eulogy-style test, and creating a ten-year plan to achieve this. Creating portfolios around the ten aspects of positivity above, in the ten emotions, is also discussed.

Alice Sommer wrote: "I was born with a very, very, good optimism. And this helps you. When you are optimistic, when you don't complain, when you look at the good side of our life, everybody loves you". *(Ms Sommer was celebrating her 107th birthday that month. She is a holocaust survivor and a musician).*

Joy, gratitude, serenity, interest, hope, pride, amusement, awe and love are listed as some of the positive emotions and the drivers, or levers that switch positivity on.

Practicing positivity makes perfect. As Ms Sommer notes, everybody will love you, and it turns out that this is an essential part of living longer and being happy about it.

More importantly, executive brain functions are powered with the desire to choose the best actions now that will ensure the best outcomes for ourselves and those we love later in time. If the executive functions receive only negatively flagged information, what exactly do we have to work with? How does motivation work when the fuel for the fire is negativity? Why do some people, in response to the good news we bring them, always point out grumpily that all is not as good as it seems to us? Perhaps they are lonely.

Jeff was a great pitcher, a major league success story. Then injury sidelined him and after two years out of the game, he finally became a free agent – otherwise known as unemployed. Going through painful therapy and with psychotherapy, he faced traditional approaches and did the best he could. However, despite improvements in his injury, he remained unable to achieve prior heights of performance and get any agents interested. When I met him, he was using psychobabble to explain where he was at. Good solid psychotherapy had forced upon him an introspection that made him miserable. "It's just that everything that comes to my mind is painted pain and black. The psych's tell me I am afraid, so I am trying to conquer my fear, without success". This young man was not afraid. We explored his biases and executive function using my toolkits, and faced negativity with some care, but his absolute failure was a vast slowness and inaccuracy on positive stimuli: therapy had turned him into a person unable to confront anything positive. He was an expert on the negative though, fast and accurate, which is where his brain had placed the resource. When we spoke about the relationship between his body and his mind, and I framed it that his body was angry with him for what he had tried to do to it, and his body did not trust him, that the relationship between body and brain was coloured by negativity, he beamed at the access this gave him to his inner world. He rapidly dived into Positivity training and rituals to change his mindset, and within a week, which was all we had, he showed marked improvement. Asking his body to forgive him, he trained body and brain to recognise and respond rapidly to the opportunities to move on, instead of being a two-year professional patient, and began to ask agents to come down and see him work. Go Jeff go!

The following chapters are for everyone, but become more important and more specific to the aging reader. Still, the rot starts early, so you have to build up a stockroom of resilience in your youth, to cover the leaner years that come. Old age certainly sucks if you have not prepared financially, but if you have not prepared in terms of your physiology and psychology, then old age can be a miserable period of decline and loss. Remember what the oldest living woman in recorded history, Jeanne Calment said when receiving and refusing an offer to restore her sight, before her death at 122 years old: I have seen enough, she said. I think she had prepared across her entire life for how it was to be as she aged. More about her elsewhere, but she had never had enough, when it came to socializing.

Many times, faced with an older, or dying person, agony is often expressed when they ask me "how did I come to be so alone?" The rot starts early there too.

Chapter Six

indigo
loneliness loves company

Many of you out there will know of Thomas Bowlby. He surfaces in the literature of the early 1930's, when he began to write on the subject of what happens to a child when early vital attachment to caregivers is broken. This means simply that when he observed children left in nursing homes to recover from contagion, or when he looked at children left alone in orphanages, he saw that their lack of secure attachment to other humans who could demonstrate permanence of emotions and contact led them to wither on the vine so to speak. Without being in the presence of caring and engaged others, they just died physically and emotionally. How do you form a self-image devoid of meaningful connections to others?

When Joiner and colleagues took their brand of self-determination to the orthopaedic wards, patients went home earlier after operations. When Sandy Forquer began to look at clinical competencies that were needed to engage mental patients in their communities after hospitalization, they spent less time coming back to hospital again, something I used in my treatment of complex needs patients, as I documented in my publication in 2001 (A neurobehavioural-informed approach to the use of clinical competencies in supporting the community based care of individuals with multi-axial diagnoses. *Australian Health Review, 24(4)*, 197-201).

Simply put, we need the presence of others to survive physically even in the absence of immediate threat to life and limb. Although the image of a lone and solitary figure may be romantic in Hollywood, replace the tough young lone gunslinger with an aging pensioner and the picture is no longer romantic. It is awfully lonely and paints a miserable, fragile, vulnerable picture. When I pointed the danger of being sedentary to one such person in a retirement facility, he noted that one of the reasons he sat around so much was that there was no one to get up for.

So Bowlby's ideas of human contact supporting the health of the children are not just true for the early years, but of the twilight ones. We understand we are gregarious creatures, and most of us, if not ill or bitter or personality disordered, will want to socialize with others as part of fun, and that is not going to wane until we are very close to wanting death.

I demonstrated years ago that social withdrawal was a totally ubiquitous response to multiple disorders of mind and body: an unhealthy person is likely to remove themselves from public contact and social intercourse, and the reverse causal link is probably true as well: when we are deprived of contact with others, we become unhealthy. (Sugarman 1999: The Phenomenology of Social Withdrawal after Traumatic Brain Injury. *Spanish Journal of Neuropsychology* (Revista Espanola de Neuropsicologia), Vol 1(4), 83-112).

John Cacioppo and William Patrick write about this in their book *Loneliness* as does Louis Cozolino in his books *The Healthy Aging Brain* and *The Neuroscience of Relationships*.

Cozolino makes mention of Madame Jeanne Calment, who lived until she was 122, the longest confirmed lifespan in history. Despite outliving just about everyone whom she knew, she lived a connected and fulfilled existence. When she went blind late in life, she opined that she had seen enough of life, and did not need an operation to restore her sight. She gave up riding her bicycle at one hundred years old, but this did not stop her attempts to get to others. When her vital connections sent her birthday greetings, she had to walk all over town to say her personal thanks to everyone who had sent kind wishes. Speaking of siloes, her nearly one kilogram of dark chocolate a week, washed down with Port Wine, certainly helped as well. You can see her quaffing these down with friends.

However, as with most humans and other primates, it was her connection to others that kept her going, hence her drive to walk the city to say thank you to her friends. Despite outliving everyone she had ever known, including Vincent Van Gogh, whom she had known as a young girl, she remained sociable and friendly, despite being widowed and having no children. As has Ms Sommer, quoted above, who both practices positivity as well as needing to be part of the social world around her, and attract people to her company.

Something about this vital connection with others guards against the exigencies of the modern world, protecting our ancient bodies and brains. For this reason, evidence exists that children who emigrate suffer worse health than those who remain behind, tied to their family and friends. For so many who emigrate to Australia or who move interstate in the USA, being connected is important, as Ma Bell used to promote in their adverts.

David Snowdon of the University of Kentucky has studied 678 members of an order of teaching nuns from the School Order of Notre Dame for the same reason. A remarkably homogenous group, they have close ties amongst their community along with eating the same wholesome meals, and receiving high levels of ongoing education while sitting less than most. They live long lives, but more importantly, despite showing remarkable signs of physical brain decay on autopsy, they typically show no symptoms of decline while alive, even when tested with sensitive neuropsychological equipment. Their death is in hospices, surrounded by like-minded colleagues and friends, some of whom may be the next generation that they personally have taught: connectedness goes from the time they join their order to the grave, with a sense this will continue beyond death in one way or the other.

By presenting the research he has found, Cozolino makes the case that high levels of social connectedness provide a solid foundation for living longer, and if it comes to a toss–up between a big cardiac bypass operation and joining a social club, there may not be much to choose between them, with a slight edge on socializing well and staying connected in retirement. Certainly being married, having family and friendship networks large and close does help the organism survive, even if the effect is to reduce stress and thus prolong life, given the dangers of cortisol and catecholamine deregulation to us physically and mentally.

Being connected to multiple groups of people tends to overcome some of the sins of daily life, namely that such vital connectedness prolongs life even in the face of obesity, smoking, drinking, low levels of exercise, and even the big killer, socioeconomic status. In contrast, social isolation, loneliness and depression add up to reduced capacity of immune systems and provide increased risk of cardiac disease.

Having other people to care for, even if you are overweight, smoking, doing little exercise, does help overcome these unhealthy aspects. Volunteering, and altruism, as I noted in the previous chapter, have their own, selfish rewards, namely a healthier immune system, fewer mood problems, and a longer life. It is said that the most selfish thing to do is live a life of selflessness. The rewards are fairly instant.

Cozolino will hold out that it was this propensity to engage and attach to others that defines the above mentioned people's resilience against the ravages of ageing. As he notes, so many of us will feel disengaged, unloved, unattractive, and certainly unneeded in later life, unless we widen our options.

What is life without close relationships? Adler is believed to have said that Freud remarked that we all need three things to thrive: somewhere to live, someone to love, and something valid to do. It's the 'someone' to love and who will return the love which Cozolino focuses on in his hypothesis. More importantly, caring for others in a directly connected way, not just paying for some kid in Africa (a good thing anyway), creates a sense of a valid and connected existence as per Freud, which pays off in terms of physical health. Anything we can do that will tell our genes we are trying to extend the life of our species, and potentially even still breed, coincides with the way we were designed to be and prolongs life. Old people in the Caucasian mountains, as with the Okinawans, live to really old age but boy, they keep on working, contributing to society, are seen as valuable by others old and young with whom they connect, and so the forces of evolution keep them healthy and going. But they work hard physically, eat well, and stay connected with the young.

This is why, when we love someone, the activation around the nucleus accumbens in the brain is surprisingly small. There is nothing urgent about loving, it keeps us quietly content. BUT: when they leave us for somewhere or someone else, loneliness threatens as a loss of vital breeding connections, so the brain activation bursts into life and we are smitten with the agony of rejection, the loss of the reward of their presence, and as we see in the elderly who are grieving the loss of their partner, this can kill. The wave of dopamine activated in the area around the accumbens is glowing red-hot; nothing matters but the return of the loved one... until the next one that we cannot live without. If there is one.

It is well accepted that when one spouse loses the other after decades of marriage, the disconnected spouse is unlikely to live much longer: however, have a look at small Greek villages at the Yaya's in black, who survive seemingly forever, connected to the family and friends who keep them alive. As I watch my friends sitting alone in the office at work and stressing out over trivial things, and alternatively see some of their wives attending gym, running around children, walking the dog, doing Zumba, I see a lot of future widows and orphans.

So Cozolino and others set out to establish the case for the brain as a social organ and an essential part of the body that both survives and thrives through stimulating interpersonal interactions. As much as young brains are built and shaped by interactions with their parent nurturers, so the caregivers in turn are served neuronal-circuit building benefits by the interaction and the meanings of these caring activities. Caring for children 24/7 or a disabled spouse may be exhausting but it fulfils the evolutionary drive, and helps overcome pain and loss in the elderly. Social connectedness is so powerful it prolongs life.

Abigail phoned me to chat about her father. He had been lingering in a local hospice for months, and quite frankly, the staff members were wondering if he was ever going to pass on. Abigail felt he was suffering, and wondered if "you did that kind of thing". So I went to see him. He certainly was not happy, in a lot of pain, and I figured he wanted to die, life was not great. But after chatting for an half hour, it was clear he had multiple concerns about Abigail, her marriage, her mood around his grandchildren, and how they all would cope without Dad and Grandad. He had been a most powerful influence, and his name was plastered all over furniture stores in the city. He was the go-to person for his wide circle of family and friends, and at ninety, he had led a full and connected life. He beat pancreatic cancer for eight years, no mean feat. Giving feedback to Abigail, she spoke to the family, and then visited her dad to speak to him and assure him all would be fine, and that she and the family would carry on without him, even though he would leave a great empty space. Leaving the hospice, Abigail got home in a half an hour to the sound of the ringing phone: he had gone.

When we are clearly past these years, and menopausal losses strike, then *voilà*, the kids have their own kids, and grandparenting begins to confer the same resilience benefits that marriage and child rearing do: longevity and wellbeing overall. If you can fool the forces of evolution into believing you are preserving the species, your genetic existence is valued and rewarded it seems. Menopause is not a passive decline, but rather a more active and orchestrated programmed cell death, with thousands of eggs still available to fertilize, but nature chooses the time to end fertility, but does not encourage any disengagement from others.

Cozolino's evidence across the lifespan begins with the current theories of why the brain ages, looking at memory, the frontal lobes, stress and the hippocampus, and of course, cognitive reserve, the phenomenon that enabled the teaching nuns to stay cogent despite their aging brain lesions.

Cognitive reserve means working constantly across the years on your brain substrate, so that you have capacity, a numbers game, a stocking up of brain cells that allows for the gradual decline by attrition of aging rather than a severe dementing decline from minimal cognitive impairment to Alzheimer's for instance. You have seen by now that the right food and the right movement help to defend that, and now you are seeing that being vitally connected and motivated to do stuff is part of building reserve as well. It's not a cure: it needs to work for years as prevention, delaying the onset of abnormal aging.

It turns out that curiosity for others may very well be the substance of a neuronal stimulus that fires the cortical tone of reserve. Cozolino looks at how the brain adapts and changes, and how it specializes across a lifetime, the connections that a lifetime of social embedded-ness brings, and how wisdom emerges. Wisdom emerges from a lifetime of being part of a huge human ecosystem, not just an observer, but vitally connected across a network: staying curious about people drives engagement. Moving frequently from place to place, or emigrating, may on the one hand harm the network, but you may develop new skills in engaging with strangers, while the internet might help sustain the past networks.

Certainly, and especially in non-literate societies, the elderly were the bearers and repositories of the wisdom of the collective groups, as in the Caucasus. This may have begun to wane along with writing and libraries; even worse, the rise of the internet and smart phones, and possibly the value of wisdom has declined with the speed at which things change, rendering in some people's minds the wisdom of our elders useless and outdated.

Most adults look to their children for advanced information about living, not to their parents, as Cozolino points out. A Native American puts it to Cozolino that without a repository for their memories, older people forget, and with nothing valued enough by others to drive the desire to pass knowledge on, slip into decline. Their wisdom dies with them as well as the emotional maturity gathered over the years, making us more afraid of the group known as the aged, to which we will all someday belong. A friend of mine remarked, looking at our teenage children, that today and tomorrow belong to them now. I found that awfully sad and nastily true for many societies. And generations of laymen are no different to academics. I note recent research making claims of being novel, claims which are deniable if I think back thirty to forty years, with forgotten research no longer reflected in their literature reviews, not what they value now, but others did it long ago. Few of us know what our Great or Great-Great Grandparents were or did. Their writings, if any, are long gone. We live in a travelling window of two or three generations of people, and those who came before disappear, for the most part. I recently looked at a video of a young and beautiful movie star, shining in her moment, and know, sadly, like Ozymandias, none will look upon her works beyond her life, and probably, give up looking long before she ages. Golden lads and lasses must, like chimney sweepers, and I guess promises, come to dust. That was Shakespeare somewhere in there.

Science advances, as our families do, one funeral at a time. We focus on a discrete part of history, and not the vast context. How lonely is it to know that even your close family will move on with their lives, and not look back too far. It is humbling.

Cozolino's next section moves to health. No surprises here: food, sleep, exercise. In terms of mindset, attributes of low neuroticism (low negativity bias) and high conscientiousness (painstaking, careful as an attribute) attend one hundred-year-old plus aged citizens, as well as extraversion and high levels of morale resulting in and from engagement with others, support from others, and the maintenance of relationships with others across time. This is just crucial to your wellbeing as any other factor, perhaps more so.

My wife is the curator of a Holocaust museum, and her favourite volunteer is a man in his nineties, a survivor of WWII, a medical doctor, a PhD, an archaeologist, the conductor of an orchestra, and so on, all in one man and now a curatorial assistant in a museum whose work is meaningful to him. Engagement with others across a lifetime thus supports physical health and mental positivity, and a reason to get up off a chair and on a bus. His engagement with his people's tragic history is his constant purpose. Why do so much? Every Jew who adds so much to the world at large attempts to prove, if it needed to be proven, how wrong it was to try to eradicate the entire nation of Jewry.

Connectedness with the purpose of your people travels down generations. French actor, singer and director Melanie Laurent is a third generation Holocaust survivor, her grandfather having survived transportation to the East. As with many '3G' survivors, she has gone into the creative arts, to contribute as the museum volunteer above has done. Unlike him, her life is not as immersed in surviving survival despite having learned to want to murder Hitler since she was five years old at her grandfather's knee. Despite this, and again in common with the connectedness of 3G with their family past, she has been involved with movies where 1) she survived a German unit's massacre of her Jewish family, another 2) where she is a nurse at a French transit camp for Jews *en route* to death, another 3) at a Jewish film festival, the Jewish daughter of a man who announces strange things... and so on. If one thinks of relatedness, connectedness, purpose, the amazing glue of motivation, you can see that large volumes of human contact are necessary to offset not only loneliness, but sustain your motivation. As with the man in the retirement home, if we are to do things, alone, then what for? For whom?

To return to Freud, we all need something valid to do. Something that resonates with our own self-image. People become nasty and decline rapidly when their disengaged life becomes invalid for them, and it is something to be avoided: social isolation kills off your mind, your brain, your emotions, and then you.

As much as we need to nurture ourselves, so we need to nurture others who engage with us, sustaining vital relationships. The importance of touch and laughter is not the province of the young alone, but of the ageing ones among us. Obviously, the presence of close relationships confers a feeling of security to the blind autonomic nervous system, so we are aware that when trouble comes we are protected to a certain extent, and at worst, we will not die alone, something that scares even younger people. And of course, in the book I am speaking of here, there is an entire chapter on grandparenting, and its value to all, as I mentioned above. This may mean that putting retirement villages right next to kindergartens might be a very good idea. Staying plugged into young people's lives is a missing and crucial part of some modern societies.

Speaking later of challenges and inclusion, Cozolino gives his predictors of cognitive health, and you will see how many emanate from Snowdon's Nun studies:

1. Education: prior and also ongoing education builds new brain tissue and connections.

2. Intellectual stimulation: novel and increasingly difficult learning daily enhances brain connections including learning novel languages.

3. Engaged lifestyle: something valid to do each day involves others in the community.

4. Strenuous activity: growth factors are released by vigorous exercise.

5. Sleep quality: too little and too much sleep predicts death and disability.

6. Low cortisol levels: keeping the cellular content of the body free of inflammation.

7. A sense of self-efficacy: what you do every day has an impact on your life, and others.

8. And of course, recovery (leisure): this is active recovery, allowing for super-compensation.

Many of the above factors are enhanced when other people are a critical element of the process. Of course, the Positive Psychologists would include the selfless sacrifice of time to others, as well as their many aspects of awe, curiosity and so on.

Cozolino advances fifty-two social things (that is, one a week in a year) that we can do, including playing with children, puppies, public displays of affection, buying an incomprehensible gadget like an iPad and getting someone young to help, and so on. I have had a look at his list, and have modified it a bit, but you will get the picture of what is in it:

- Play with children or socialize with younger people wherever possible.

- Learning something new from someone new, each day.

- Pick a good cause, learn about it, and then join people

who will fight for it.

- Engage in public displays of affection, as do politician's wives.

- Go to a new restaurant, eat something unusual.

- Keep your hearing and eyesight well controlled and working.

- Travel, and stay at a youth hostel and hear what young people have to say.

- Buy a new gadget and get a young person to show you how it works.

- Vacation in small, foreign places where you are forced to meet people.

- Join a group that plays something, like cards or a sport.

- Find a young person to mentor in what you are passionate about.

- Teach at a learning center near you.

- Take advanced driving or sporting courses.

- Go to the ethnic side of the supermarket and get someone to show you how to cook stuff that is foreign to you.

- If you are engaged with people with a negative outlook, dump them!

- Engage with people who are positive.

- Write a song and sing it in public, go to Karaoke clubs.

- Rediscover your curiosity in strangers and what they do.

- If you have always taken care of others, get someone to take care of you.

- If you have always taken, give to others, work for charity.

- Hang out at the library, animal shelter, pavement coffee shop.

- Talk to strangers, lots of them.

- Take classes in subjects you have never studied before.

- Take dance lessons.

- Go back to school.

- Write a letter to old friends you are no longer in contact with.

- Track old friends on the internet. Arrange a future with them.

- Wear an odd shirt or hat that attracts attention, or badges or barefoot shoes.

- Buy a really cute puppy, walk it around the beach, the neighborhood, anywhere.

- Name your pets strange names, something to talk about to strangers.

- Carry out three random good deeds for total strangers each week.

- Volunteer for a soup kitchen.

- Volunteer to help kids at Summer Camp or a homework group.

- Watch live sporting events.

- Haunt second hand, new book shops and antique fairs.

- Go to motor shows and motor auctions.

- Enrol in cooking courses or debate or speech societies.

- Take an adult education course in a cool subject to talk about to others, e.g. film.

- Do another degree on a campus and hang out with students and tutoring groups.

- Take up photography and move around a lot outdoors, do portraits of strangers and send them copies on the internet.

- Chew chewing gum to control breath odor; launder clothing well, keep windows open, burn essential oils, eat carefully, maintain hygiene, make your body and house fresh and clean. Stay lean and look sporty, trim your hair close.

- Take up pretend smoking and allow strangers to talk you out of it.

- Make up your own socializing drivers and for heaven's sake:

- Read Cozolino's book.

You can integrate a desire to socialize more with the motivation structure I gave you above, as you can with any aspect of movement, or nutrition, for instance: try this with the socialization gaols using the goals suggested by Cozolino above or make up your own:

Health Change Contract Socializing More!!

1. Set one goal for Socializing and Laughing for each page of your Change Contract:

    _____

2. List three of YOUR most IMPORTANT, meaningful reasons to laugh more and socialize more:

    a) _____

    b) _____

    c) _____

3. To build your CONFIDENCE, list small, meaningful steps to your goals:

    Where I am now: (A) _____

    Step 1 _____

    Step 2 _____

    Step 3 _____

    Step 4 _____

    Step 5 _____

And any other small steps until **B: My Goal is reached**.

4. Which three signs show your READINESS to begin laughing and socializing more immediately?

a) _____

b) _____

c) _____

I am reminded of a nice Japanese story. A lonely man approaches a psychologist who recommends he purchase a dog to walk with in the park each night so he avoids the lonely spot in front of the TV. Soon enough, while sitting in the park with his dog, he meets another dog owner, and leaving the dog at home alone, spends time each night with her and her friends, getting home later and later each night, the dog pawing at the door, dying to get out, becoming increasingly lonely and frustrated. This goes on more and more, until one night, he comes home late, and finds that he has left the kitchen door open. So....

No, no, no, you are wrong! The dog is still there, but the cat has gone. Cats just will not put up with that kind of neglect. Cats are selfish. So are young people: they have to have a reason to be around you, and so you have to continue to be interesting, eat and dress well, keep your body and mind clean and stimulated, and forget the old days: there are great lessons from the old days, but hell, they were second rate compared to being young now!

So the time to build resilience is now, in your thirties or earlier. Being fat and unhealthy and lonely as a kid leads to the same situation as an adult. No one will deny that the real reason for what we are as humans is the presence of other people and our vital connections to them. As much as self-acceptance is vital, even as a human shape which does not conform to photoshopped needs to accept who and what they are, the opinion of others and acceptance by others is crucial too. With the majority of people in Western societies headed for obesity, acceptance for being larger than necessarily dictated by nature is increasing, and political correctness is making it easier for oversized people to accept their appearance. If that were all there was to say about it, I would shut up.

But: fat, lonely, bullied kids have fatty liver risks, 'diabesity' risks, shortened lifespan, and a host of other ills to come. They cannot serve their country in time of war. They are unable to comfortably sit in a coach or in an airliner. Now they need new chairs, bigger coffins, and bigger graves to be dug. Acceptance of their lot in a non-discriminatory society without prejudice is desirable, but leaving them be and accepting the numbers in children and adults as inevitable is not on, and will bring most countries and their medical and defence systems to their knees.

Despite it being a modern world, the race will always go to the fittest and the strongest and the prettiest and the brightest, or all in combination. A fit, but fat person is still entirely possible, but unfit is unwise, not just unattractive by Barbie standards. The loneliness of being outside of modern, photoshopped norms, in a society that values most its youthful sporting and showbiz celebrities, means that a vast majority of our population has role models they can never emulate in any real way. This has led, in pathological cases, to stalking of celebrities by damaged people, by many fantasies of a connection that does not exist, reading, looking, wanting, what is part of the new leadership of the world. This builds more loneliness, more isolation. Self-acceptance has nothing to do with a passive approach to your body and brain, accepting your life is not an excuse for accepting how it got to be that way, as a static end point. It really is about change. Doing everything in your power to make the best you can out of what you have, is the true meaning of success.

My grandparents, perhaps yours, depending where you came from, told me one of the most open roads to happiness was "knowing your place in the world". This was a form of Cockney humbleness and acceptance that said airs and graces were no way to go forward. Stoically accept your lot in life, and who you are, and silly to expect too much else. A strange thought to today's motivational speakers, and the parents of atonal kids headed for auditions for American Idol. Not a good idea to look at the TV screen and dream of things you will never, ever aspire to. You just will never belong to them, or they to you. Barney the Dinosaur sings that you are special. You are not special, but you are unique, and that is not a bad thing. There is a place for you in the world, and there are no real global forces conspiring against you which you should heed, and remain with what you have, not wanting what you cannot have. The question is how much you are prepared to engage with the world and fight for a place in keeping with your talent, work ethic, and a bit of luck. Successful people all have stories, and so many come from nothing to something that way.

This is why competitive work with good money is better than volunteer work in healing disability for instance. If age is not to be a disabling condition, we have to be with, around, and connected to others in vital ways, and maintain our space in the world.

We know that caring for others helps us live longer: women who give birth after forty are more than four times as likely to live to a hundred. Male apes and monkeys who share childrearing live longer than other species, which do not. Having a grandmother around at age two helps children survive better into adulthood.

Because social contact helps regulate our stress responses, in fact the entire hypothalamic-pituitary-adrenal system, the calmer, safer and more supportive our social world, the better we regulate resilience and hence are healthier, and can compete better and with less.

Loneliness itself has huge health risks. The authors Cacioppo and Patrick are not alone in considering the value of belonging, or relatedness, given that Louis Cozolino and others have already added to the literature on the subject.

As the world tries to deal with living longer but less healthily, one of the situations which we are urged to avoid is the loneliness which may accompany old age, and, which may accompany a whole host of illnesses, as Cozolino and others suggest.

At the coffee shop along the high street in my road is a daily visitor, a resident really, Jan-Luca by name. At age seventy-six, and unaware of the day and date, he engages with just anyone passing by, or certainly sitting to drink coffee. He asserts that he has no idea how he came to be lonely at his age. His antidote, driven by a need to consort with others, is to sit at the pavement café every day. At five p.m., as the shutters roll down, he passes through the pedestrian crossing to his apartment, only to emerge and repeat his day the next day, like Groundhog Day. He says if he did not, he would just shrivel up. Every passer-by gets a greeting, especially if they have a dog: even the younger girls do not mind the creepy attention; he is after all, Italian. As I write this, he is consigned to a nursing home, where hopefully there will be others to talk to. However, it will be hard for him. He told me he dreads the day there will be no passers-by who are young, pretty, with cute dogs to walk past. To engage with, and for a second or two, pretend he is one of them.

Humans are desperate it seems to form individual and group liaisons with multiple others. Certainly, it seems we evolved language and social systems to do this, as we lost our protective jaws and claws and probably our four-legged locomotion and became vulnerable as loners. When we are ill or depressed, or damaged in some way, we tend to withdraw socially and lick our wounds. And that means we are alone and vulnerable, with a higher risk of death or disability.

Social systems, even in fairly ancient looking societies such as the 11 000 year old ¡Kung or Khoisan in the Kalahari Desert of Southern Africa appear to be fairly typical of such agrarian societies. Their hunting and living are cooperative, and it appears the capacity of the females to share themselves in dallying with others is also promoted, allowing for gossip and other entertainments. Breast feeding is on demand until five years old or more, children are carried in a sling for about 1500 miles a year, and the ¡Kung carry on pretty much as they did before. Being stingy is a serious offence, giving is everything: this does not create a Utopia, as the ¡Kung murder rate amongst themselves is higher than the USA per capita (female dallying is a serious pastime). Nevertheless, their tight knit and altruistic society underpins what we all value: other people, service, community.

The authors explore in depth the interplay of three essential factors in the 'sting' of loneliness or social exclusion. Most of us have the nasty experience of being chosen last in the playground or classroom or at a dance, or some other place, as the sting of social exclusion is understood by all, when it violates our self-image especially. Choose Me!

While it may no longer mean certain death, as it does in the African savannah, social exclusion can certainly drive people to despair, depression or even suicide. Our level of vulnerability to social disconnection is mentioned by many motivational scientists, speaking of the drive that is increased by a sense of social connectedness, a sense of valid relatedness, not just mastery, when we contemplate change.

Loneliness begins finally to disrupt our ability to self-regulate our emotions and also our social cognitions. It is a two-way street, with social separateness and dislocated emotions and cognition in turn leading to further social disconnectedness and further self-fulfilling negative thoughts and actions.

This higher sensitivity to events and feelings, at the same time with less accuracy in viewing life, creates a vortex, which is difficult to escape.

This also leads to other behaviours: for instance, loneliness leads us to seek and enjoy unhealthy food, even if we rate the food poorly in terms of taste and satisfaction: this helps us understand why the stereotyped TV character, recently dumped by a lover or disappointed by a parent, is destined to appear onscreen with a tub of double chocolate something or the other, and eats it all.

As Baumeister found with cookie experiments, it is clear that lonelier adults tend to seek out and eat fattier foods, and if loneliness is measured by a scale, for each standard deviation off the mean lonely people consume about 2.5% more calories from fat. The upper layers of our brain, comprising the neocortex, are not thus immune to the influences from the 'troops' below, and when they get lonely, behaviour and cognition change and we adopt less valuable behaviours like comfort eating. Cooking for one person is inevitably poor, and living on a single income will enhance unhealthy choices.

Research connected to loneliness is spurred on by the changes in our society. We have demonstrably fewer close persons to discuss important issues with, despite social networking sites that allow us to connect widely but superficially with others. Average households are smaller, and increasingly run by a single parent.

In 2000, twenty-seven million people lived alone in the USA, 36% of them under the age of sixty-five, estimated this year to rise to twenty-nine million, an increase in more than 30% since 1980....and of course we are getting fatter, for reasons the authors make clear. One is reminded of what Hobbes suggested life might have been like without the social contract that guided our culture and laws: solitary, poor, nasty, brutish and short... I wonder if that will still emerge as the dominant life for many with social media becoming the single most growing form of socialization... but at a distance?

Experts in loneliness have to ask why loneliness promotes so much wear and tear on the body-brain system, so as to occasion illness.

Social isolation on its own has been shown to be on a par with other risk factors, such as hypertension, obesity, sedentary behaviour, and smoking as risk factors for illness and early death. One would imagine this is a behavioural issue, but the effect sizes are too large.

Social class, as examined in the famous Whitehall British Service study, confers many risks, as do lack of social connectedness itself and even obesity clusters in social classes. Less education, less money, not only at the bottom end of the ladder, with imbalances in effort and reward and low levels of control in one's working life, act as independent predictors of cardiovascular events even when all other variables are controlled for. Lack of self-efficacy, or even a sense of low self-efficacy, is deadly.

Loneliness and health, say the authors above, have five causal pathways. **Health behaviours** (executive control is compromised by loneliness), **exposure to stress and life events** (again, perceived control is an issue) so then **perceived stress and coping** are influenced as well, the **physiological response to stress** such as the allostatic load of loneliness is higher (the effects on the nervous system), and **rest and recuperation** are also impacted by loneliness.

Drawing on genetic evidence, part two of the Loneliness book plays on the words 'selfish genes', as put forward by Dawkins, and the authors then set out to show how there is more than just social influence at play here, more than just a skewing of our self-image by comparison to those around us. This discussion involves the intra-subjective nature of our emotional social development, and the way we respond to subtle cues and outright rejections.

The book by Cacioppo and Patrick, a must read for all of you out there, finally provides an **EASE** approach to social connectedness: to address social isolation, it may be necessary to.

1. **E**xtend yourself

2. Develop an **A**ction plan

3. **S**elect more promising relationships, and

4. Adopt an **E**xpect-the-best philosophy.

Connectedness, Relatedness, Purpose:

Cozolino however has more to offer than the Loneliness authors: his book on *The Neuroscience of Human Relationships* goes further in more ways than I have given above:

If you thought the title was about boy meets girl, it's not, it's about mum meets baby and baby meets mum in a reciprocal bonding and attachment relationship, and the neuronal plastic adaptations that follow, enabling adult interactions with the social environment. As the Russian founder of Neuropsychology, Alexander Luria wrote more than half a century ago, socialisation ties the cortical knots in our brains that make up who we are in our culture: in short, our self-image in relation to others.

Cozolino writes that it is the power of being with others that shapes our brains. By attachment, in its reciprocity, we bind to another and establish ourselves in terms of our 'self'. Psychotherapy has long paid attention to bonding, since Bowlby, who I have mentioned a few times before: (see my review *Treating Attachment Disorders: From Theory to Therapy,* 1999 – **Google: Metapsychology, Roy Sugarman 2286**).

Elizabeth Gould, a scientist at Princeton, has shown that the brain indeed is responsive to the environment, and I do mean response in terms of literally growing or declining in the face of environmental factors, which would include the quality of social life.

Louis Cozolino has written before about the neuroscience of psychotherapy (see *The Neuroscience of Psychotherapy: Building and Rebuilding the Human Brain,* 2002 – **Google: Metapsychology, Roy Sugarman 1836**).

In a somewhat similar vein, he takes on another psychosocial encounter, but one which is natural, and less contrived. Cozolino evaluates how we live in our relationships, with an influence on the subjective experience of being with others from our perspective, and also how we are created in terms of these encounters, with our evolution as social creatures inextricably bound up with our biology.

Essentially, this was the first time an integrated approach took hold, as Bowlby and others are clear on the relation between body and brain and environment: it is the absolute fine exemplar of the validity of the field.

We survive because initially we have others to engage with in real ways, such as the mother as our primary environment, driven by socially-based parenting drives to protect us and later instruct us for personal as well as altruistic, group reasons. In many ways the drives that nurture are non-selfish, enhancing the wellbeing and continuity of the group, or immediate species, as the positive psychologists have shown. Self-image is thus relationally forged.

The second chapter refers to an evolving brain, namely one that is not born with any real maturity, and thus takes time to evolve with the creature into an independent self-image. An interesting fact is expressed about the whites of our eyes, which evolved so that others could see where we were looking, as opposed to those with unicolour eyes, predators, whose prey needed to not see where they were looking.

Other methods that evolved enable us to demonstrate to others that we are not just blank tablets for socialization to write on, include blushing and pupil dilation.

The social changes in adolescence (accompanied by increases in white matter and decreases in grey matter), also challenge our connectedness and how we socialize. Cozolino relates this to the changes in social interaction that make demands of the teenager.

We experience socialization at the brain level, but the benefits are overwhelmingly physical, in terms of building resilience.

Use the measures above to manage your contact with the outside world, and accept how valuable contact with others really is, especially the contacts you make in the service of others. Engagement, certainly at an emotional level, does depend on how you engage verbally with other people.

Effective Communication: good people ask, they do not tell.

This is about building and maintaining relationships, and understanding other people.

You may think that working with others is about talking: it isn't. It's about listening, effectively listening and making sure you have heard what was being communicated. This is not the same as ordinary listening, but is rather 'reflective' listening. Reflective listening helps people engage with you, as they realize by your actions that:

1. What they say is important to you.
2. You find things about them that you like.
3. You are a scarce resource which is available to them.
4. The relationship is a warm, supportive, and positive one.
5. You can be helpful in clarifying their thinking process.

You may think this might be difficult to achieve, but these skills can be taught through simple practical exercises rather like batting practice. We throw things at you: you hit them back at us. You are the expert in you, but now, you have to become expert about others: practical solutions are the best after all.

Reflective listening is what psychologists use in their conversations with patients. An acronym you might like to use is the OARS approach from Miller and Rollnick's work on motivational interviewing.

O = Open Ended Questions

We need to get others to do the talking, to make the compelling arguments for change or collaboration with you. One way to do this is to avoid getting simple Yes or No answers when we question them. An open-ended question gets them to examine their thoughts more closely. Asking a child how their day at school was elicits "Fine!" and that is usually the end of that conversation. A more open ended question is designed to get a fuller answer out of the other person, to get them chatting to you and hence more engaged in the relationship.

A = Affirmations

When the conversation is on the go, you will need to make contact with the other person emotionally, getting them to realize that you see positive values being demonstrated by what they are saying. We have to make others feel good about themselves to keep them engaged. This means reflecting on what they have answered to (above), and finding something positive to say about them, so they feel the emotional connection.

R = Reflection

People engage well when we acknowledge the emotions underlying what they are saying, a form of acknowledgment of their roles and position in the world, in a positive way. Reflection is a way of checking with them that the emotions behind what they are saying are being heard accurately. This confirms for them that they have an empathic audience, and by definition, an engaged one.

S = Summary

Following the process above, we take time to summarise what we have heard so far, and in doing so we pick out selectively the good, the positive, the valuable aspects about what we have heard from them, while showing that we are checking to see that we got all their important messages correctly. We choose only about three things during a single summary and then follow that up with an open ended question, beginning the cycle again. It is rather like gathering a bouquet of what they have said and offering them the flowers of their wisdom back again. The flowers you see as the best aspects of them. This shows that we regard what they have said as being important, so much so we want to check with them that each pearl of wisdom has been noted correctly: as I offered though, three or four main points are enough, or this can be irritating if we reflect on everything they have said.

The OARS Approach to Better Social Engagement: a deeper dive

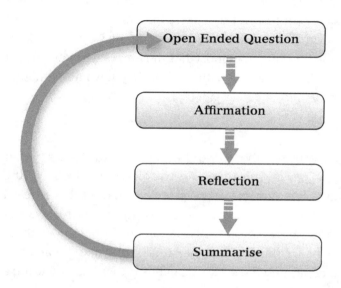

Open Ended Questions

The last thing you want here is a monosyllabic reply, such as *No, Yes, Fine, Whatever.* Let us take the scenario of someone talking on the phone.

"How was your day at work?" This could be responded to with a single word. What about a more open ended question? Think of one of these, for instance:

- So tell me all the good things and all the not so good things that happened at work today, start with the not so good okay...?

- So how did your morning go with all the things you had scheduled, tell me what happened with each…

- I wasn't with you this morning; so tell me what happened on all fronts…

- Hey, I haven't seen you for a while, so catch me up on your projects at work…

As you can see, it is difficult to respond with a *Yes* or *No* or *Nothing* to these questions. The questions ask for information, but go further in that they demonstrate that you are REALLY interested, not just being polite. Your **A-R-S** that follows the **O** will be consistent with this message.

Affirmations

As noted before, you have to find something positive to say to the person. Let's say the response to a question above went as follows:

"Not too bad, but a lot of things went wrong, little things that I had to get my head around. The boss asks a lot of questions about things I have no access to so I have to scurry around to get them"

A possible response to this, focused on making them feel a positive emotion about themselves could be:

- I really admire the fact you keep cool and avoid losing it with him.

- It's great that you can think on your feet and never admit you have no idea what he is on about.

- You have done well to cope with that situation for so long, I have no idea how you manage!

- You never let him get you down; you just have a way to get around his sabotage.

In this way, you avoid giving advice, but show you see the valuable and positive things about their bad situation, not making it worse, supporting them, and showing them the up side of their struggles with life. People like people who like them, as Dale Carnegie said.

Reflection

Empathy is such a vital part of relationships, and reflective listening is another big aspect that cements empathy in the relationship. Carl Rogers was the great champion of this approach. By reflecting emotional content, you place the relationship in a warm, close category, encouraging people to relax and be themselves around you. It's not easy though, especially if you do not want to be seen as insincere, superficial, or soppy. Never ever use the phrase: "You feel…" by the way, it's not a good intro. You have to be real, so batting practice is necessary.

Have a go at interpreting these sentences. In the previous example, you heard what the person said about their boss in response to your open ended question. Think of the emotion in their sentence, "Not too bad, but a lot of things went wrong, little things that I had to get my head around. The boss asks a lot of questions about things I do not get access to so I have to scurry around to get them". What emotions were there? Take the sentence bit by bit.

A typical reply after the affirmation response might include the following reflections. Look at how many ways we can say to someone, I heard what you said, and let me check how it all felt to you, so we can connect on a deeper level of understanding:

- That must be so frustrating for you.

- Little things that like can be sooo infuriating!

- You must work under continued pressure, no?

- So only little things, but they do mount up do they not?

- It must be hard to be peppered with questions all the time.

- Getting your head around so much detail must wear you down.

- I am sure the lack of access must make you feel it's all too hard...

- I think you are so strong when you say, "not too bad"; it must be really hard for you to be positive.

- So exhausting to scurry around, it would be nice if things could be more accessible.

Summarizing

Now that you have got them to this point, take time to reflect on what they have told you so far, emphasizing what you think was important in what you heard. In order to make them feel and act more positively, emphasize in your summary what you want them to focus on. Keep your summary to the three main points you want to make. For instance:

"Thinking back on what you said, it's amazing that despite the position, your boss puts you in, you just seem to be constantly trying to move forward, harvesting your energy, meeting the demands. That's such a sign of strength to me; I really admire that in you".

And of course, you close with an Open Ended Question to start the cycle again:

"So tell me what keeps you going in terms of your attitude?"

In closing, here is a quick look at a simple conversation: watch out for the O-A-R-S and then O here:

"Hi"

O – "Hi, what kind of things happened this week?"

"I've been so busy with various things"

A – "You have always been the industrious type, got a lot done?"

"Nothing much"

R – "It's so frustrating when you put your heart and soul into things, and yet so little outcome"

"That's for sure…." silence"

S – " So despite you chasing your tail all over the place, you feel disappointed at seemingly getting nowhere: (and here is the O) what kind of flags need to pop up before you feel you have gotten somewhere?

Now remember one final thing: People learn by DOING. So get out there and practice batting **O**, **A**, **R** and **S** with someone, and ask them afterwards how they felt during your conversation. Chances are they felt great.

Chapter Seven

VIOLET

down time is actually productive, recovery is everything

Noleen *was getting on in years but approached me with two problems: she was fatigued, and was losing her temper...a lot. She was now beginning to see her memory was not as good and was worried about dementia. She was 'cut' (high muscle definition), not an ounce of fat, a great figure, and loved by many, with a large family and friendship group. Money was not an issue, as her husband had done well. Diet was near perfect. After some misdiagnosis and a lot of medical investigations, it became plain her cortisol levels were off the chart, and she was becoming insulin resistant. Determined to overcome this, she worked out more often at the gym, ate differently, took on a personal trainer. It got worse. She would get up later in the mornings, always feeling fatigued. When I pointed out to her that her exercise regime of seven days a week was building up impressive cortisol and noradrenaline, she was shocked: as with many, she did not realise her* *hectic physical training, work and socializing schedule left her no down time, no recovery. She asserted she was happy and never stressed, but it was clear she was. Forced to comply, and train only three, sometimes four days a week, she noted her memory and angry outbursts improved. With massage, meditation, Tai Chi, stretching and mobilizing, and less high intensity workouts, she began to feel a lot better. Quiet times were introduced when she just chilled with a book.*

Although at Athletes Performance we teach that movement, nutrition, mindset are the first three pillars of a great athlete, there is a fourth pillar that we should never forget: recovery. Recovery is the time when brain and body utilize the growth hormones produced by the load we place on the body, and build new tissue, compensating for anticipated future strains with growth and resilience.

Overtraining in its various formats in our modern lives is a crucial source of dysfunction. We simply have to allocate compensatory activities and not go at it like lunatics. Many men, successful and hardworking, leave their wives playing card games with friends as widows. These women may not be left grieving and wearing black, but might, in reality, now be freed from children and household duties, free to travel and enjoy life. Many never saw their men much anyway.

But there are strange things we do each day that we never think of as strange.

For instance, after an (exhausting) day of sitting down in front of a computer, we sit in traffic for an hour or two, or on a train, and then we flop into a chair, and do some more sitting. Then we go lie down and sleep. As I have pointed out before, this is not part of how we are designed to be: we are built to move.

We go work out hard at the gym each day, not realising that our bodies are in worse shape when we finish than they were when we started: we have to take time to recover actively to make the workout do its job of enhancing our health.

Essentially however, we can endure longer than any other creature, namely we can hydrate and feed as we move and thus go on endlessly. Tim Noakes, and other researchers dating back to the 1920's, believe that only the limiting effect of the brain switches us off, and theoretically, we can carry on using our muscles until a central governor in the brain tells us we are on the brink of injury, so we then feel fatigued and stop.

The mere action of sitting down is not a good recovery strategy, certainly not as a form of recovery after sitting down the entire day. Recovery means active recovery. Walking, stretching, mobilizing, hydrating, massaging, using vibration plates, doing some cognitive challenge, which is totally unique compared to the work we do, e.g. learning a new language or a new discipline, like the archaeology of the rain forest or physics.

So we need to recover from working. Sitting, focused intently on a screen in a triple-flexed position is harmful and so the term 'recovery' means to rehabilitate your body after damage has been done by doing repair work, regeneration work. We also have to recover from another major stressor, namely, exercise.

Recovery strategies have to be built into your daily and preferably hourly, working and resting life.

Ever wondered why you get sick when you begin an annual vacation? No longer under the threat that daily working and driving activity brings, the body resorts to being thrifty. The immune system, if not engaged in proper work, is a very expensive machine to run in terms of metabolic demand. Thus, when the body husbands its resource, the immune system is allowed to drop out of action. It is somewhat like going from DefCon 5 to DefCon 2, in nuclear war terms.

As I have mentioned, exercise is a stressor, keeps the body aligned with defending itself, and thus keeps the edge going with high levels of cortisol. Movement, such as Tai Chi is recovery, as Scarmeas and others have shown.

My mother-in-law is a classic case in this regard. Even at seventy plus, she keeps working as a real estate agent, up early, gets to bed late, watches what she eats, gets to Pilates often. At the end of a hectic year, she goes off to an island paradise where she sinks into the chaise lounge and with a sigh of relief does nothing but rest, sleep, lie and watch the sea, idyllic. At the end of ten days, she bends over to caress a grandchild, and goes home two days later in a wheelchair, having put her back 'out', something that does not happen during her working year. Passive recovery is dangerous, for body and brain. Her son, on the other hand, goes on holiday and does not sit down for a second, scuba, windsurf, surfing, gym, boxing, jogging, anything but sit. Heading for forty, he is built like an athlete.

As the little family scenario advises, a default strategy for your life should not include lazy relaxing or retirement: these are distinctly fatal in many cases.

The take home message here is that frantic workouts, on the one hand, as with Noleen, and sitting on your rear end such as my mother in law on holiday, or particularly those who work in an office or driving a car for most part of their day, are two sides to a very unhealthy coin. Either extreme is likely to end in disability.

Recovery, regeneration, rehabilitation, are ACTIVE processes

Gerald was in his mid-thirties, doing well at work, going to the health club to work out each day, happy to get his body pumped up after a whole day in the car or in his busy office. After the bodybuilding routine with his personal trainer, Gerald dashed home to his wife's exemplary cooking (she was a chef before kids came along), a glass of red, and then flopping in front of the TV where he inevitably dozed off. One night, his wife noted his breathing was unusual: then to her horror, it stopped. She waited for the snort, or snore that often followed, but nothing happened, then she noted his lips were blue and his eyes were open slits. Throwing him to the floor, she shouted to her neighbour to call the emergency number, and began what she had learned in the restaurant, doing hands-only CPR. Given their proximity to the local fire department, two minutes later Gerald was being defibrillated, after which he was transported, conscious, to the emergency room.

If you look carefully at the scenario above, the only recovery really built into his life was flopping on the sofa after a rich meal and alcohol, and then dragging himself off to bed. It took a very short time to convince him to not work out seven days a week, or sit for long, unbroken hours, or change his diet, or more correctly, change his eating behaviour, and understand how overtrained and stressful his life had incrementally become without him knowing it. Speaking to him, it was clear his father was dead at fifty-three, his grandfather at fifty-eight, and they had lived the same life as he was now attempting.

Heart Rate Variability Training

The press recently has documented two particular soccer players, one in England and one in Italy who dropped dead on the field during a game. Later on, a Norwegian Olympian swimmer died in Arizona. Then a seventeen year old teenager we know locally collapsed on the soccer field.

I note in fact there have been dozens in recorded history, young men in their prime, and not only in soccer or swimming but also in other games, such as Basketball, marathons, and so on. How can such 'healthy' young men experience sudden death? People die in marathons and on the sports field every year. These people are not actually 'healthy', but often have some underlying heart disease, very commonly in cardiac terms these are undetected arrhythmias, or a sudden loss of the rhythm that keeps the heart beating and the brain healthy.

We need to learn a bit about this beating of the heart and recovery, because there is something awesome and of great value to recovery and building resilience here, thanks to the work of Dick Gevirtz from San Diego, Paul Lehrer and others.

In terms of how we as humans are put together, the tenth cranial nerve is an interesting one. Many researchers believe that the lower third of the Vagus (#10) has evolved unusually in humans.

What this means is that the brain, the Vagus, the lungs, blood pressure regulation, etc., are all tied together in the following way:

When we breathe in, the feedback action of using our lungs produces a steady, metronomic heartbeat, and the dominance of the sympathetic nervous system. This means that on inspiration, our flight-fight-freeze mechanism is active, readying us for combat or flight or great stillness to avoid or combat our enemies. You will notice that at a sudden loud noise, you gasp a breath in, and a whole host of metabolic stuff happens which readies you to face danger. So overall, this is a necessary sequence of events that protect us, but not healthy in the long term, to keep firing this mechanism. Under prolonged stress, the whole system, as Hans Selye pointed out, can lose its specificity and adaptability, namely lose the precise focus for real danger, e.g. sabre tooth tigers or traffic police, and respond to traffic, queues at the supermarket and so on as if we were in mortal danger. This may often be accompanied by hyperventilation with some light headedness, and in a vulnerable individual, panic. Chronic hyperventilation (and most people breathe up to twenty-two breaths per minute) may also result in night time awakening when cortisol climbs, with a thudding regular heart rate that seems to not vary for a while.

Not that being immune to the effects of stress is healthy either. Interestingly, there is research to show that soldiers with advanced combat training, namely Special Forces training, have very regular metronomic heartbeats, with high levels of Neuropeptide Y as well, so they are built to cope with combat stress and do not freak out as I might. Whilst most of us will finish a day of combat with little Neuropeptide Y to speak of, these soldiers will end with normal levels, having started with much higher levels.

However, the downside for these soldiers, should they survive combat is a reduced life expectancy later in life. It turns out that this heartbeat profile where each beat is exactly the same distance in time from the next, is not conducive to living a long life, which is what we are all trying to do (if you are interested in survival training and this phenomenon, read Charles Morgan and his colleagues works in *Biological Psychiatry 2000, Vol 47; Mind Wars: Brain science and the military in the 21st Century.* J D Moreno, Bellevue Literary Press, May 2012).

Now, on the other hand, breathing out has a different action, part of Respiratory Sinus Arrhythmia, as the Vagus nerve exerts a braking phenomenon on the heart rate. When we breathe out, the heart rate peaks vary from each other in time, perhaps one hundred milliseconds each, and this results in parasympathetic dominance, the 'rest and digest' branch of the autonomic nervous system. It turns out that if you can work out which breathing rate will give you the best beat to beat variation, called the resonant frequency (see Paul Lehrer's work), then you can optimise the action of the parasympathetic nuclei in the brain, and also reach the calmest state to enhance recovery. Breathing rates around four breaths per minute, but not lower, and probably up to six breaths per minute, will do the job nicely it seems.

So the more time you spend breathing out rather than breathing in, the better you have tuned your autonomic system to attend to its recovery, as represented by a preference for parasympathetic activity rather than sympathetic, noradrenergic activity as with Noleen. Stress during daily, modern existence keeps you in sympathetic mode, leading to distortion of the purpose of this part of the nervous system. If it is true that you have to play as hard as you work, and I would pretty much agree with that in terms of recovery, then you need equal time in parasympathetic mode, which is the ANS version of a relaxing holiday, which drops your vigilant responses to what in reality are non-life threatening events.

So it turns out that the maximal extent of HRV you can manage is associated with calmness and health across a wide variety of issues, including blood pH and blood pressure recovery.

The steady metronomic beat of the sympathetic dominance, which is probably where most of us spend our time, like Gerald did above, is not healthy in the long term, and is associated with a higher risk of death.

Even in brain injury, for instance, poor HRV levels are associated with poor outcomes.

In athletes, poor HRV is a marker of still being in recovery from prior effortful training, and a sign to wait before training hard again, or risk a failure to thrive and flourish.

HRV is thus a great tool for recovery.

A quick way to bring this into your life is to try for three minute bursts during the day, accumulating up to twenty minutes a day of this kind of breathing where you maximise the time spent breathing out, and increase your CO_2 levels as well, which is calming, especially for those prone to anxiety and worry.

An important point here: this is not to be done to **avoid** panic when it hits; rather, it is a form of training. Using it during a panic attack might be counterproductive and promote avoidance of noxious stimuli: think of this as inoculation, a way of building resilience and assisting physical and mental recovery and not an attempt to avoid unpleasant anxiety or panic at the time, but rather to avoid getting into that state at all later.

As much as I recommend you move around often during a sedentary day, I also recommend using HRV training during the day. You can do it anywhere, in the car, in the bathroom, in the elevator.

The quick method is known as 6:4:10. In this way, you breathe in for a count of 6, hold it for 4, and breathe out for 10 or more. This can be counting in seconds if you like, but that would be three breaths a minute, which most of us find hard to do.

So breathing in this way can help inoculate you from the deleterious effects of stress, aid your general mood and health, guard against cardiac events, generate calming Alpha activity in the brain and assist your transition to sleep. It will also regulate your blood pressure and pH of your blood, all of which is helpful.

You can prepare for stressful meetings at work, or headed for the stadium if you are an athlete, or combat as a soldier. It helps you focus, and assists you in dropping your blood pressure or returning your heartbeat to a resting rate after exercise.

I must emphasise that depression has huge cardiac risks, independent of other factors. HRV training is essential to help minimise this risk, as depression and poor HRV and low vagal tone are associated with death in such patients, and of course bad sleep hygiene.

Pain is another great target for HRV training.

By now, you will think I am going over the top about HRV. But the Vagus is a major conduit of body brain activity and regulation, and so altering sympathovagal noradrenergic activity is a really useful target for a host of conditions, which are impacted by this system. This would include heart, mood, anxiety, worry, blood sugar, blood pressure, acidity, negativity bias, working memory, delta, theta and alpha activity, lateral prefrontal cortex and amygdala volume, positive mood and a host of other factors. Have a look at any Google search and you will see what I mean. A few references for you can be found at the back of the book in Addendum A.

Let's see what a day with recovery might mean, in general terms for someone who wants to recover on an hour by hour basis during the day:

1. Sleep more than seven and a half hours a night, but not more than nine.

2. Wake up and do three minutes of HRV 6:4:10 breathing.

3. Do a gratitude ritual for a few minutes.

4. Leave the bed immediately after awakening; do not sleep in as there is evidence that this may induce unhelpful sleepy brain waves that do not clear during the day.

5. Do some stretching and mobilizers: you can find plenty on YouTube, and your personal trainer or physical therapist will have more for you.

6. Do some planks, push-ups and other wake up drills.

7. Have a cold shower, gradually decreasing the hot after washing until under pure cold water.

8. Eat a breakfast of whole grain, with some honey and cinnamon, provided you can tolerate gluten, or otherwise spelt bread with avocado on it, or grilled vegetables if you are so inclined.

9. Swallow some fish oil tablets, Vitamin D, Co-Enzyme Q10, Selenium, Vitamin B Complex, and avoid antioxidant pills otherwise, discuss other necessary supplements if you have a family doctor; get blood tests to see what you need in terms of supplements.

10. Hydrate a lot: you might not have had liquids for twelve hours or more.

11. Take a fruit snack with you to work. Get some coffee or green tea in you, without sugar or milk.

12. Do Heart Rate Variability training for three minutes wherever and whenever possible.

13. Drink 300ml per 10kg of body weight per day, keeping your urine clear, more if you exercise or are female (350ml). In USA terms, this is half your pound body weight, but using ounces as the measure, so 100 lb.=50 Oz water per day, more if necessary: do not use plastic water bottles, even if they are bisphenol free, they pollute you and the environment: tap water in a glass or tin bottle will do nicely.

14. Take the stairs to work.

15. If you commute on a train, stand the whole way holding on to a handrail, letting your legs, knees slightly bent, do the work as the train moves.

16. Set your timer for forty-five minutes each hour. Stand up, do a complex mobilizer-dynamic stretch, walk to the bathroom on another floor, set your computer to print on a station far away.

17. Eat some Omega-3 rich food, like almonds or other nuts.

18. Eat a light lunch of salad and proteins, with lots of avocado, olive oil, seeds, nuts; and some carbs like noodles or bread, especially before exercise where the carbs go to muscle, not to the liver as fat.

19. Take a walk in direct sunshine after lunch.

20. Every second day, work out at the gym. If you do not have one, go to the park and do some interval training.

Run or walk until breathless, then slowly until entirely recovered. Do this for twenty minutes at least; running on the spot with arms pumping, for ten seconds at a stretch, with ten-twenty seconds rest in between sets.

21. Every other day, do recovery at the park or beach, walking briskly, mobilizing, stretching, very light weights if you must use them. TRX, Vipr's, medicine balls, all good.

22. If you drive home, do not make up time with your telephone, rather listen to music, and avoid the news like the plague: it's too much over which you have no control.

23. When you get home, say Hi, go and shower, then walk the dog.

24. Cook with your partner, starting from fresh produce and grass fed/free range meats. Eat a light, grilled meal, with plenty of plant oil, but only cook with oils with a high flashpoint, like avocado oil, not olive oil for instance unless you control the temperature.

25. Have a bit of dark chocolate and red wine. I said only a bit.

26. Do not watch the news: usually it is negative and distressing.

27. Watch some comedy on the TV while standing and doing the ironing.

28. Listen to music rather than TV, dance with your partner.

29. Avoid sitting, apart from eating time.

30. Make sure the TV is off when you are eating.

31. Avoid TV and Computers or other light sources in your visual field within ninety minutes of your bed time; get ready for bed when not tired: when sleepy, go straight to a dark quiet cool bed.

32. Do some stretching before bed. Tense and relax tight muscles.

33. Do up to twenty minutes HRV training a day, especially while awaiting sleep.

34. Write all your thoughts about the day and what must be done the next day on a dump pad. If you wake up thinking about anything during the night, write it down on the dump pad.

35. Practice some mindfulness and Positivity stuff, as well as HRV.

36. When you are sleepy, switch off the light.

37. As I said, sleepiness usually comes in ninety-minute bursts. Do not start preparing for bed during a sleepy feeling, otherwise it may be gone by the time you hit the hay. Plan your switch off time for when the tiredness hits.

38. Every week, try schedule a massage. Buy a massage stick and a foam roller. Look up their use on the internet.

39. Find time to meditate wherever possible, do mindfulness rituals.

40. Schedule dates with your partner at restaurants that serve healthy organic food.

41. Learn to make your own red wine, preservative free, it is not that hard!

42. Book socializing times well in advance to keep up with old friends.

43. Volunteer at a charity organization.

44. Phone family, avoid negative friends, unless you can do something for them, and they take your advice.

45. Get to beaches, public places and pools, enjoy cold water and use ice on insect stings, sore muscles, and suck on ice for heartburn or gastritis.

46. Learn to dance.

47. Buy a dog, or rather two, so the one can keep the other company: confide in your dogs a lot.

48. Be affectionate wherever appropriate.

49. Read inspiration works or watch videos of Mother Theresa and others doing good things for people. TED. com is a great place to start.

50. Rescript bad dreams into good ones, just before falling asleep again using HRV.

51. If you wake up at three to four a.m., urinate, hydrate, and do some HRV training to fall asleep.

Here is a good workout for recovery from worry if you find yourself regularly worrying about something:

Problem Solving Worksheet: use this whenever you find a problem is making you negative.

1. Nature of the problem

   _____

   _____

   _____

2. On a scale of 0-10, where 0 is 'not poor' and 10 is equivalent to the death of a child or loved one, how bad is this problem?

   0-1-2-3-4-5-6-7-8-9-10

3. If this problem is not resolved, what is the worst that can happen?

   _____

   _____

   _____

4. If you accept (3), then what can you do to make this bad outcome, better?

   _____

   _____

5. Who can help you with this problem? List them in order of both value to you and their capacity to help you in effective ways without blame or scolding you.

_____

_____

_____

6. Look at all the things you will definitely lose if (3) happens: is any of these something you love and cannot live without? If none, then revisit (2) and downgrade the disaster score by half.

7. Looking at what you will lose if (3) happens: can all of these things be undone by money? If yes, then revisit (2) and downgrade the disaster score by half.

8. Go forward 5 years after (3). What will your life look like if you make this bad thing better (4)?

_____

_____

_____

_____

_____

_____

9. Solving the problem:
    (a) Simulate the possible outcomes and your solutions, and write them down
    (b) have you had a similar problem before, or has someone else you know had similar? If so, see if this works by simulating as before
    (c) brainstorm with others about simulated outcomes
    (d) remember to fragment the steps taken in (4) at micro goals, so the main problem is not so overwhelmingly negative
    (e) can you use totally different scenarios for solutions to this problem
    (f) look at what caused the problem in the first place, can this be undone
    (g) find solutions, then try to make them fail in simulation, choose ones that are hardest to beat
    (h) use a GROW model:
    G = what is your goal?
    R = the reality of how far in means and ends you are from the goal. How many mini-goals should be achieved?
    O = what are the obstacles to each mini-goal?
    W= way forward for tackling each obstacle to each mini-goal
    (i) use PDCA model:
    P = plan each mini goal
    D = take action on each
    C = check your progress each step of way
    A = act on each failure to progress in C and do a GROW PDCA on each

(j) use Eight Disciplines if you can in a team setting, or a group of friends :
D1 = use the team
D2 = define the problem
D3 = take small actions based on mini-goals
D4 = identify root causes
D5 = take big actions based on the big goal of resolution
D6 = implement and validate
D7 = modify your systems so the problem does not recur
D8 = reward yourself and people that helped.

You will see the commonalities of all these approaches. Firstly, identify the problem, how bad it really is, how it got that way, what has to be done if the worst happens, set small goals that are not overwhelming, test them out in a simulated way using input from others, each failure should be treated as a problem in itself, for each micro goal that does not work, take it one step at a time. Above all else, do not be overwhelmed by focusing on the big picture, just focus on the baby steps. And finally, be active: passive worrying is the enemy of your resilience!

So recovery is not about trying to escape stress.

Stress is always with us. Sustained stress is a problem, and wreaks much less damage on our system if we break it up into small chunks, hence my instruction to move and break up what you are doing every forty-five minutes or so. In this way, if you graphically represented Stress versus Strain across your day, instead of a constant, escalating curve, you would see a step-wise graph ending far lower than the one without any breaks. Strain is a measure of the load on your system causing damage or fatigue:

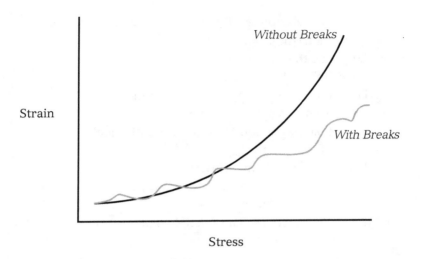

So taking frequent breaks is the same as going on holiday multiple times a year instead of a single break at the end.

Another good idea is to formulate a strategy for when you are in a crisis of any kind. The worst time to have to work out a strategy is when you are in the middle of a crisis. The Problem Solving Worksheet above is one such way of dealing with the crisis.

This is why I rely so much on HRV training: its like taking a week-long holiday for three minutes at a time.

Recovery and the immune system:

Out of all the systems in your body, by far the most expensive and intricate to maintain is the immune system. This is why you often get sick when you slow down and go on holiday after a long working year. Another group prone to infection is the peak athlete, or people who go to gym often and are fitness fanatics with little recovery time. Not washing your hands before and after gym doesn't help you. Your body, if stretched, will not find the time and energy to keep the immune system coping well when demands are being made, often excessively, on the body and brain at the gym. Worse, during extreme exercise, the body may turn to the cartilege and bone of the joints to find the amino acids it needs during heavy workouts in civilians who are being silly, training like peak athletes or combat marines. Having blood tests at the doctor might not show up exactly what is needed in terms of nutrition, as this focuses on the plasma of the blood, not the cells of the body. Cellular analysis is available, and various groups supply micronutrients based on these assays of cellular tissue. Thus, even if you are a real gym fanatic and blood and guts runner or trainer, you have to be careful about attending to recovery and making sure your body and brain can sustain both a healthy immune system as well as peak performance. Look at Lance Armstrong and other athletes who are young and fit when they are diagnosed with cancer: huge demands on the body and brain need to be scaffolded with judicious use of carbohydrate, hydration, protein, fats, and micronutrients. Otherwise, injury and illness are not far away. Athletes use illicit drugs and steroids to speed up recovery, and thus train more often and harder. Armstrong, with all his accolades, is now disgraced forever. Winning cannot be everything forever.

It is worth repeating: Down time is productive time, not wasted opportunity, and has to be incorporated into what you do, in the workplace or on the sportsfield, so as to allow for the body and brain to keep up with demand, and secondly, build resilience against increased usage.

Active recovery, such as walking, yoga, Tai Chi, playing golf, or swimming slowly, as well as more passive recovery, e.g. massage, meditation, study, all will have benefits, in contrast to hammering your body six days a week at work and at the gym. Nothing healthy or good will happen until you recover, and during recovery is where body and brain build for the future as a new form or more resilient form of you.

> *Without recovery, all you are doing is working too hard, and you will pay the price.*

Sleep

So, it is natural to sleep eight hours or so a night? Actually, it's a fairly new invention. Seriously.

Lets first look at sleep, which occurs in stages:

Stage 1 is a drowsy, relaxed state between being awake and sleeping – breathing slows, muscles relax, heart rate drops. Stage 2 is slightly deeper sleep – you may feel awake and this means that, on many nights, you may be asleep and not know it. Stage 3 and Stage 4, or Deep Sleep – it is very hard to wake up from Deep Sleep because this is when there is the lowest amount of activity in your body. After Deep Sleep, we go back to Stage 2 for a few minutes, and then enter Dream Sleep – also called REM (rapid eye movement) sleep – which, as its name suggests, is when you dream. In a full sleep cycle, a person goes through all the stages of sleep from one to four, then back down through stages three and two, before entering dream sleep.

As I alluded to above, a growing body of evidence from both science and history suggests that the eight-hour sleep may be unnatural.

Psychiatrist Thomas Wehr conducted an experiment in the early 1990's in which a group of people were plunged into darkness for fourteen hours every day for a month. By the fourth week the subjects slept first for four hours, then woke for one or two hours before falling into a second four-hour sleep. This is not a hugely new phenomenon, in fact, it was how we always slept.

Historical references describe a first sleep which began about two hours after dusk, followed by a waking period of one or two hours and then a second sleep. During this waking period people were quite active. They often got up, went to the toilet or smoked tobacco and some even visited neighbours. Most people stayed in bed, read, wrote and often prayed. Countless prayer manuals from the late 15th Century offered special prayers for the hours in between sleeps. And these hours weren't entirely solitary – people often chatted to bed-fellows or had sex. A doctor's manual from 16th Century France even advised couples that the best time to conceive was not at the end of a long day's labour but "after the first sleep", when "they have more enjoyment" and "do it better".

It was simply too dangerous to go outside into the dark, which was the habitat of thieves, footpads, prostitutes, and homeless people. The rich stayed at home with their candles.

References to the first and second sleep however started to disappear during the late 17th Century. By the 1920s the idea of a first and second sleep had receded entirely from our social consciousness: the answer lies in the industrial revolution and the advent of real lighting, taking back the streets from the criminals and the poor.

Initially, improvements in street lighting, domestic lighting and a surge in coffee houses – which were sometimes open all night, started to change the face of our natural sleep culture. As the night became a place for legitimate activity and as that activity increased, the length of time people could dedicate to rest diminished and settled into the sleep we now think of, one unbroken sleep, right through the ultradian, cortisol cycling.

Associations with night before the 17th Century were not positive. The night was a place populated by people of disrepute and drunks, as noted above. Even the wealthy, who could afford candlelight, had better things to spend their money on than that. There was no prestige or social value associated with staying up all night at that time. The Reformation and counter-Reformation saw Protestants and Catholics become accustomed to holding secret services at night, during periods of persecution. Respectable people became accustomed to exploiting the hours of darkness.

With the advent of street lighting, socialising at night began to filter down through the classes. In 1667, Paris, the City of Light, became the first city in the world to light its streets, using wax candles in glass lamps. It was followed by Lille in the same year and Amsterdam two years later, where a much more efficient oil-powered lamp was developed. London didn't join their ranks until 1684.

Again, our ancient bodies in the modern world were to have the most vital aspect of recovery, namely sleep, modified and processed. By the end of the century, more than fifty of Europe's major towns and cities were lit at night. Night became fashionable and spending hours lying in bed was considered a waste of productive time and the industrial revolution intensified that attitude towards efficiency awareness by leaps and bounds. Strong evidence of this shifting attitude is contained in a medical journal from 1829 which urged parents to force their children out of a pattern of first and second sleep.

Today, most people seem to have adapted quite well to the eight-hour sleep. Many sleeping problems may have roots in the human body's natural preference for segmented sleep as well as the ubiquity of artificial light, smart phone and computer and tablet screens included in the light that dominates the dark.

Middle Insomnia first appears in literature at the end of the 19th Century, at the same time as accounts of segmented sleep disappear. For most of evolution we slept a certain way. Waking up during the night is part of normal human physiology.

Sleeping too much is also no good. Researchers find not only increased mortality in those that sleep too much, but include a risk of metabolic syndromes in those who sleep more than eight hours habitually. You can imagine that waking up and moving from your prone sleeping pose after four hours was helpful in reducing such risks. Sleeping too little has other risks, including some behavioural ones, such as becoming unethical in your decision making in business. Sleep deprivation mimics physical stress on the body, and is connected to being overweight or obese. Sleep too much, sleep too little, in a million person study by Kripke in *The Archives of General Psychiatry* in 1979, predicted a host of mortal illnesses.

When we miss a night of sleep, our bodies make up for it by going through a more intense bout of slow-wave activity the next night. Slow-wave activity occurs during non-REM sleep, and involves large parts of the brain going into a synchronized rhythm, or oscillation. Rebound, intense slow-wave activity is essential for restoring our ability to focus and pay attention. Sleeping pills inhibit slow-wave activity. So taking a sleeping pill on the next night following a bout of insomnia might not be as effective as it needs to be, or so says an article in *The Journal of Neuroscience*, February 4, 2009.

Surveys conducted by *The National Sleep Foundation* reveal that at least forty million Americans suffer from over seventy different sleep disorders and sixty percent of adults report having sleep problems a few nights a week or more. Most of those with these problems go undiagnosed and untreated. More than forty percent of adults experience daytime sleepiness severe enough to interfere with their daily activities at least a few days each month; twenty percent reporting problem fatigue a few days a week or more; sixty-nine percent of children experience one or more sleep problems a few nights or more during a week; and in Australia, according to *The Sydney Morning Herald*, Seventy percent of Sydneysiders say they are tired every day.

Irritability, moodiness and disinhibition are some of the first signs a person experiences from lack of sleep. If a sleep-deprived person doesn't sleep after the initial signs, the person may start to experience apathy, slowed speech and flattened emotional responses, impaired memory and an inability to be novel or multitask. As a person gets to the point of falling asleep, he or she will fall into micro sleeps (five to ten seconds) that cause lapses in attention, nod off while doing an activity like driving or reading and then finally experience hypnagogic hallucinations, the beginning of REM sleep (you can have a look at Dinges writing in *Sleep, Sleepiness and Performance, 1991*). In general, most healthy adults are now prone to experience sixteen hours of wakefulness and need an average of eight hours sleep a night. However, some individuals are able to function without sleepiness or drowsiness after as little as six hours sleep. Others can't perform at their peak unless they've slept ten hours. Contrary to common myth, the need for sleep doesn't decline with age but the ability to sleep for six to eight hours at one time may be reduced. (Van Dongen & Dinges, *Principles & Practice of Sleep Medicine*, 2000).

What causes sleep problems?

Psychologists and other scientists who study the causes of sleep disorders have shown that such problems can directly or indirectly be tied to abnormalities in the following systems:

Physiological Systems

- Brain and nervous system

- Cardiovascular system

- Metabolic system

- Immune system

Furthermore, unhealthy conditions, disorders and diseases can also cause sleep problems, including:

- Pathological sleepiness, insomnia and accidents

- Hypertension and elevated cardiovascular risks (MI, stroke)

- Emotional disorders (depression, bipolar disorder)

- Obesity; metabolic syndrome and diabetes

- Alcohol and drug abuse (Dinges,2004)

Groups that are at particular risk for sleep deprivation include night shift workers, physicians (average sleep = 6.5 hours a day; residents = 5 hours a day), truck drivers, parents and teenagers. (*American Academy of Sleep Medicine and National Heart, Lung and Blood Institute Working Group on Problem Sleepiness*, 1997).

Sleepiness takes a toll on effective decision making. In experiments it was found that alert people are very sensitive to the amount of work they need to do to finish tasks and understand the risk of losing their money if they fail. Sleepy subjects choose to quit tasks prematurely or they risk losing everything by trying to finish the task for more money even when it was one hundred percent likely that they would be unable to finish the tasks. For more, you can read further on what Dr. Timothy Roehrs, the Director of research at the Sleep Disorders and Research Center at Henry Ford Hospital in Detroit wrote in the August 2004 issue of the journal *'Sleep'*.

According to the Department of Transportation (DOT) in the USA, one to four percent of all highway crashes are due to sleepiness, especially in rural areas and four percent of these crashes are fatal. Risk factors for drowsy driving crashes include:

Late night/early morning driving, patients with untreated excessive sleepiness, people who obtain six or fewer hours of sleep per day, young adult males, commercial truck drivers, night shift workers, and frighteningly for us all, medical residents after their shifts.

According to leading sleep researchers, there are techniques to combat common sleep problems:

- Keep a regular sleep/wake schedule, routine is king here.

- Avoid drinking or eating caffeine four to six hours before bed and minimize daytime use, even if you tolerate it well, as the quality of sleep may be disturbed.

- Avoid cigarette smoke, especially near bedtime or if you awake in the night, it is too stimulating.

- Avoid alcohol and heavy meals before sleep, as again, quality of sleep is affected.

- Get regular exercise, early morning, not late at night, for cortisol reasons again.

- Minimize noise, light and excessive hot and cold temperatures where you sleep, cold is better than heat and about 60°F or 16°C is about right. You wouldn't store wine that hot would you?

- Develop a regular bed time and go to bed at the same time each night.

- Try and wake up without an alarm clock, hide the clock from sight!

- Attempt to go to bed earlier every night for certain period; this will ensure that you're getting enough sleep.

- Keep away from light sources such as phones, tablets, computers, TV. Turn the brightness down to minimum for nightime use.

- Avoid absorbing TV shows, if you have to watch before bed.

- Put a dump pad next to your bed, for the bright ideas that keep you awake, but are gone by tomorrow.

- And watch out for ultradian rhythms

Resources

Measure and manage your sleep: have a look at the Zeo Sleep Manager,
http://www.myzeo.com/sleep/

National Sleep Foundation
http://www.sleepfoundation.org/

American Academy of Sleep Medicine
http://www.aasmnet.org/

American Insomnia Association
http://www.americaninsomniaassociation.org/

Sleep Research Society
http://www.sleepresearchsociety.org/

NIH National Center for Sleep Disorders Research
http://www.nhlbi.nih.gov/sleep

Victorian Government Sleep Resource:
http://www.betterhealth.vic.gov.au/bhcv2/bhcarticles.nsf/pages/Sleep_problems_insomnia

Sleep Health Foundation:
http://www.sleephealthfoundation.org.au/pdfs/Insomnia.pdf

Getting good at getting to sleep is vital for recovery.

So that kind of does it for the seven areas of the wellbeing rainbow. So now what?

Chapter Eight

gold
the golden pot at the end of the rainbow

So now you put this book down, yawn and go back to your unhealthy modern life. Why?

1. **I'm not sick**: well, not something your doctor might note now, today, but the rot starts long before you know of it, or show clinical symptoms. Alzheimer's and cholesterol and arterial and cardiac issues hide for decades and grow gradually. Responding only when you are sick is not the best default strategy for building resilience. This will engage you with doctors, and as you age you will become one of the polypharmacy patients cuing up at the window for your pile of pills. Becoming disabled will lead to 70% of you becoming depressed, and requiring more pills. When you have some illness manifesting, it is usually noticed too late to reverse. You start to die in your thirties, and only realise this in your seventies: do

something now, build resilience NOW. Try not to add to the statistics of people in their thirties and forties who are claiming disability. What on earth will you look like at seventy? Now, do stuff, and do it NOW.

2. **I have no time**: little things make a big difference and DO NOT absorb time. Do little things that add up to big things. You will have to find time for doctors, medicine, chemotherapy, surgery, recovery, and find huge funding for this later on. So you will find time now and be happy in the future that you started NOW. If you have no time now, do you really believe you will find time at seventy? It will be way, way too late by then. There is a door to vitality open now, not so much tomorrow, and someday, it can close entirely, and for ever.

3. **I'll start tomorrow**: No you probably will not. Intelligent people procrastinate. In a week or a month henceforth, will you be happy you did NOTHING today or tomorrow, or will you already be a week down the road toward building resilience, and already feeling better? Failure to act now is not rewarding.

4. **Where do I start**? Start with setting goals for each week from now for six weeks, choosing one thing out of each chapter from one to seven. Set a day during that week when you do that one thing, such as seeing your doctor, or taking the dog or kid to the park for a run around the tree game of catch, or buy a glass water bottle for your desk at work. Every six weeks revise what you are doing by adding another one action a week. In twelve weeks, you will be doing twelve healthy things a day, and well

on your way to living life longer and loving it. Recruit a close friend or partner, and swear an oath to them. Better. Give a friend a bank-guaranteed cashiers cheque for $500 to be cashed and taken if you DO NOT adhere to what you are promising to do. This will work in the short term. If you are rich, give them $5000.

5. **I hate healthy food**! Try the 80-20 rule, then the 90-10 rule a few weeks later. This means getting most of your calories from healthy food, some from the fun stuff like alcohol and chocolate. Get to 99-1 and you are THE MAN! More importantly, although some food might taste horrible to you, you can make it taste better by reading recipes, e.g. for broccoli or cauliflower, and making the twenty percent or ten percent the grilled Parmesan and paprika you add to the grilled vegetables. Use an excuse, e.g. well Parmesan cheese is full of tryptophan which boosts serotonin to help you sleep, like turkey for instance, and paprika helps protect against stomach ulcers, so grill that onto the broccoli, which by the way is a good anti-cancer agent for smokers. Red Peppers have a lot of bronchodilating chemicals like capsicaine that help asthma, so help yourself that way as well. Tomatoes are really healthy cooked, so do them that way, and put them on top of your GRASS-fed beef or lamb to enhance the Omega 3 in those meats. If you miss cold cuts, do your own, buy a whole fillet steak and grill it rare with no salt, and use that thinly sliced as a replacement for bought cold cuts. If you hate fish, add 3000mg of fish oil caps into your diet each day. Nothing wrong with whole cream milk or butter, remember, you could use avocado instead,

but avoid human processing issues, low fat stuff (means high sugar), no sugar stuff (means high fat) and avoid cereals for breakfast which have whole grain boasting, but when you look on the sides of the pack only seventy-five percent is oats etc, the rest is sugar or something evil! Oh, you hate oatmeal? Buy the quick version, 100% oat version, cook for two minutes with milk, add syrup and tons of cinnamon (good for Alzheimer's, so's coffee by the way, and coconut oil), and cook for another one minute, delicious! Not too much fruit, okay, and do not juice it, just liquidize it in a blender: do not ditch the fibre. You love salt? Ditch it and use herbs, spices, black pepper etc, and you will learn to not need added salt, there is enough in the bread. You WILL get used to good food and develop a taste for vegetables and soon will puke if someone offers you unhealthy options.....we hope. Follow a Mediterranean or Paleo diet, no 'health' food or preponderance of rabbit food, if you must.

6. **I hate my personal trainer, and PT's in general**. First of all, change gyms! If you can chat to the trainer, if they are approachable, ask them to do more regeneration and recovery work with you on alternate days, and see if any in the gym are Effective Movement Trained, or know how to use Vipr's, CoreTex, Kettle Bells, Functional Movement, Intelligent Movement, PowerPlates, TRX, Battle Ropes, Sleds and so on. These are much more fun and healthy, and involve a host of work in the gym you will find more engaging. Many trainers do this outdoors in parks and beaches, and that is even more fun. Try Zumba, Tai Chi, Qi Kung, ballroom dance, etc.

If you train yourself, remember to add mobilizers in between each and every robust exercise, to get those fascia moving smoothly, and avoid injury and overtraining. Recovery is King.

You have to remember this dear reader:

That I am only visiting your life in this book, you have to live it.

You are the expert in you, and so only you can make the compelling argument as to why you should live an integrated life, and in so doing, live life longer and love it.

Change is hard, so change on your own terms, for your own reasons, and in so doing, adopt healthy behaviours that are meaningful to you. Do not try to comply with the guidance or wishes of others.

Little things make a big difference: changing small aspects of your life will make a huge difference.

Recover as hard as you train or work: active down time is not wasted time, it is essential.

The rot starts early, so start while you are young, and even if you are healthy now, that is relative and may not last, the damage you are doing now may cost you later, in spades.

Modern food and liquids may not be fuel, but slow poison: eat low Human Interference.

Eat a wide range of food, and avoid faddy diets unless absolutely necessary.

Do not waste money on supplements unless indicated by a professional: it's just expensive urine.

Eat your antioxidants, as opposed to the taking them in pill form.

Stay moving your whole life, including holidays, or pay the price later in life for being sedentary.

Break up any required sitting with movement of all your joints, and mobilize and stretch.

When your body is worked, you can work your brain, as they are one and the same.

Do not listen to me – listen to you. I am not a sage on any stage, nor a guru. I am part scientist and part friend, here to help you adopt healthy change not just comply with my guidance. However, think of this below, now you have read this book:

You are an ancient body in a modern world. So are your children. Do you really want to outlive them, and continue to stop each day at the service station store and buy them salt, sugar, caffeine and rancid oil products to stuff into and inflame their bodies? Then let them go home and sit in a triple flexed position? Is that not child abuse? And look at what you are eating, and how much time you are sitting. Do you really want to leave your partner and your children alone, and miss out?

Why would you not want to be a better version of all the good things you are?

If all of this now makes you feel uncomfortable, then I have done my job. For it is what you do, that makes a difference: not me.

Roy Sugarman PhD

www.roysugarman.com

Sydney, Australia 2012

Dr Roy Sugarman

Addendum A

Heart Rate Variability References

Baumert, M., Brechtel, L. Lock, J., Hermsdorf, M., Wolff, R., Baier, V., Voss, A., 2006. *Heart Rate Variability, Blood Pressure Variability, and Baroreflex Sensitivity in Overtrained Athletes*. Clinical Journal of Sport Medicine, 16(5),412-417.

Bernardi, L., Porta, C., Spicuzza, L., Bellwon, J., Spadacini, G., Frey, A.W., Yeung, L.Y.C., Sanderson, J.E., Pedretti, R., Tramarin, R. 2002. *Slow Breathing Increases Arterial Baroreflex Sensitivity in Patients With Chronic Heart Failure.* Circulation 105, 143-145.

Berntson, G.G., Cacioppo, J.T., Quigley, K.S. 1993. *Respiratory sinus arrhythmia autonomic origins, physiological mechanisms, and psychophysical implications.* Psychophysiology 30, 183-196.

Berntson, G.G., Cacioppo, J.T. 2004. *Heart Rate Variability: Stress and Psychiatric Conditions.* In: Marek Malik, A. John Camm (eds), Dynamic Electrocardiography, Blackwell Publishing, Futura Publishing, Elmsford, New York.

Berntson, G.G., Norman, G.J., Hawkley, L.C., Cacioppo, J.T. 2008. *Cardiac autonomic balance versus cardiac regulatory capacity.* Psychophysiology 45(4), 643-52.

Billman, G.E., Dujardin, J.P. 1990. *Dynamic changes in cardiac vagal tone as measured by time-series analysis.* Am J Physiol. 258, H896-H902.

Birkhofer, A., Schmidt, G., Förstl, H. 2005. *Heart and brain – the influence of psychiatric disorders and their therapy on the heart rate variability.* Fortschr. Neurol. Psychiatr. 73, 192-205.

Booij, L., Swenne, C.A., Brosschot, J.F., Haffmans, P.M., Thayer, J.F., Van der Does, A.J. 2006. *Tryptophan depletion affects heart rate variability and impulsivity in remitted depressed patients with a history of suicidal ideation.* Biol Psychiatry 60, 507-514.

Britton, A., Shipley, M., Malik, M., Hnatkova, K., Hemingway, H., Marmot, M. 2007. *Changes in heart rate and heart rate variability over time in middle-aged men and women in the general population* (from the Whitehall II Cohort Study). Am. J. Cardiol. 100, 524-527.

Bonnemeier, H., Richard, G., Potratz, J., Wiegand, U.K., Brandes, A., Kluge, N., Katus, H.A. 2003. *Circadian profile of cardiac autonomic nervous modulation in healthy subjects: differing effects of aging and gender on heart rate variability.* J Cardiovasc. Electrophysiol. 14, 791-799.

Carney, R.M., Blumenthal, J.A., Freedland, K.E., Stein, P.K., Howells, W.B., Berkman, L.F., Watkins, L.L., Czajkowski, S.M., Hayano, J., Domitrovich, P.P., Jaffe, A.S. 2005. *Low heart rate variability and the effect of depression on post-myocardial infarction mortality.* Arch. Intern. Med. 165, 1486–1491.

Carpeggiani, C., Emdin, M., Bonaguidi, F., Landi, P., Michelassi, C., Trivella, M.G., Macerata, A., L'Abbate, A. 2005. *Personality traits and heart rate variability predict long-term cardiac mortality after myocardial infarction.* Eur. Heart J. 26, 1612-1617.

DeGuire, S., Gevirtz, R., Kawahara, Y., Maguire,W. 1992. *Hyperventilation syndrome and the assessment of treatment for functional cardiac symptoms.* American Journal of Cardiology, 70(6), 673–677.

Depue, R.A., Kleiman, R.M., 1979. *Free cortisol as a peripheral index of control vulnerability to major forms of polar depressive disorders.* In: Depue, R.A. (Ed.), In the Psychobiology of Depressive Disorders. Academic press, New York.

Dietrich, A., Riese, H., Sondeijker, F.E., Greaves-Lord, K., van Roon, A.M., Ormel, J., Neeleman, J., Rosmalen, J.G. 2007. *Externalizing and internalizing problems in relation to autonomic function: a population-based study in preadolescents.* J. Am. Acad. Child Adolesc. Psychiatry 46, 378-386.

Fagard, R.H., Pardaens, K., Staessen, J.A. 1999. *Influence of demographic, anthropometric and lifestyle characteristics on heart rate and its variability in the population.* J. Hypertens. 17, 1589-1599.

Gianaros, P.J., Van Der Veen, F.M., Jennings, J.R. 2004. *Regional cerebral blood flow correlates with heart period and high-frequency heart period variability during working-memory tasks: Implications for the cortical and subcortical regulation of cardiac autonomic activity.* Psychophysiology 41, 521-530.

Glassman, A.H., Shapiro, P.A., 1998. *Depression and the course of coronary artery disease.* Am. J. Psychiatry 155, 4–11.

Glassman, A.H., Bigger, J.T., Gaffney, M., Van Zyl, L.T. 2007. *Heart rate variability in acute coronary syndrome patients with major depression: influence of sertraline and mood improvement.* Arch. Gen. Psychiatry 64(9), 1025-31.

Gockel, M., Lindholm, H., Niemistö, L., Hurri, H. 2008. *Perceived disability, but not pain is connected with autonomic nervous function among patients with chronic low back pain.* J. Rehabil. Med. 40(5), 355-358.

Gorman, J.M., Sloan, R.P. 2000. *Heart rate variability in depressive and anxiety disorders.* Am. Heart J. 140, 77-83.

Hansen, A.L., Johnsen, B.H., Thayer, J.F. 2003. *Vagal influence on working memory and attention. Int. J. Psychophysiol.* 48, 263-274.

Hassett, A.L., Radvanski, D.C., Vaschillo, E.G., Vaschillo, B., Sigal, L.H., Karavidas, M.K., Buyske, S., Lehrer, P.M. 2007. *A pilot study of the efficacy of heart rate variability (HRV) biofeedback in patients with fibromyalgia.* Appl. Psychophysiol. Biofeedback 32, 1-10.

Hemingway, H., Shipley, M., Brunner, E., Britton, A., Malik, M., Marmot, M. 2005. *Does autonomic function link social position to coronary risk? The Whitehall II study.* Circulation 111, 3071-3077.

Herbs, D., Gervirtz, R.N., Jacobs, D. 1994. *The effect of heart rate pattern biofeedback for the treatment of essential hypertension. Biofeedback and Self-Regulation,* 19(3), 281.

Jackson, S.A., Csikszentmihalyi, M.C. 1999. *Flow in Sports: The Keys to Optimal Experiences and Performances.* Champaign, IL: Human Kinetics.

Karavidas, M.K., Lehrer, P.M., Vaschillo, E., Vaschillo, B., Marin, H., Buyske, S., Malinovsky, I., Radvanski, D., Hassett, A. 2007. *Preliminary results of an open label study of heart rate variability biofeedback for the treatment of major depression.* Appl Psychophysiol Biofeedback 32(1), 19-30.

Karavidas, M.K. 2008. *Heart Rate Variability Biofeedback for Major Depression.* Biofeedback 36(1), 18-21.

Kitzlerová, E., Anders, M. 2007. *The role of some new factors in the pathophysiology of depression and cardiovascular disease: overview of recent research.* Neuro. Endocrinol. Lett. 28, 832-840.

Kleiger, R.E., Stein, P.K., Bosner, M.S., Rottman, J.N. 1992. *Time domain measurements of heart rate variability.* Cardiology Clinics, 10, 487-498.

Lehrer, P.M., Vaschillo, E., Vaschillo, B. 2000. *Resonant frequency biofeedback training to increase cardiac variability: rationale and manual for training.* Appl Psychophysiol Biofeedback 25(3), 177-91.

Lehrer, P.M., Vaschillo, E., Vaschillo, B., Lu, S., Eckberg, D.L., Edelberg, R., Shih, W.J., Lin, Y., Kuusela, T.A., Tahvanainen, K.U.O., Hamer, R.M. 2003. *Heart Rate Variability Biofeedback Increases Baroreflex Gain and Peak Expiratory Flow.* Psychosomatic Medicine 65, 796-805.

Lehrer, P. (2007). *Biofeedback training to increase heart rate variability.* In R.W. Paul Lehrer, Wes Sime (Ed.), Principles and practice of Stress Management (3rd ed.). New York: Guilford Press.

Logier, R., Jeanne, M., Tavernier, B., De Jonckheere, J. 2006. *Pain/analgesia evaluation using heart rate variability analysis.* Conf. Proc. IEEE Eng. Med. Biol. Soc. 1, 4303-4306.

Lucini, D., Riva, S., Pizzinelli, P., Pagani, M. 2007. *Stress management at the worksite: reversal of symptoms profile and cardiovascular dysregulation.* Hypertension 49, 291-7.

Maestri, R., Pinna, G.D., Porta, A., Balocchi, R., Sassi, R., Signorini, M.G., Dudziak, M., Raczak, G. 2007. *Assessing nonlinear properties of heart rate variability from short-term recordings: are these measurements reliable?* Physiol. Meas. 28, 1067-1077.

Massana, J., Lopez Risueno, J. A., Masana, G., Marcos, T., Gonzalez, L., & Otero, A. 2001. *Subtyping of panic disorder patients with bradycardia.* European Psychiatry, 16(2), 109–114.

Mezzacappa E, Tremblay RE, Kindlon D, Saul JP, Arseneault L, Seguin J, Pihl RO, Earls F, *Anxiety, antisocial behavior, and heart rate regulation in adolescent males,* J Child Psychol. Psychiatry 38:457-469, 1997.

Monami, M., Marchionni, N. 2007. *Psychological disorders and cardiovascular diseases.* G. Ital. Cardiol. (Rome) 8, 335-348.

Moldofsky, H. 1994. *Chronobiological influences on fibromyalgia syndrome: Theoretical and therapeutic implications.* Baillieres Clinical Rheumatology, 8(4), 801–810.

Murialdo, G., Casu, M., Falchero, M., Brugnolo, A., Patrone, V., Cerro, P.F., Ameri,P., Andraghetti, G., Briatore, L., Copello, F., Cordera, R., Rodriguez, G., Ferro, A.M. 2007. *Alterations in the autonomic control of heart rate variability in patients with anorexia or bulimia nervosa: correlations between sympathovagal activity, clinical features, and leptin levels.* J. Endocrinol. Invest. 30(5), 356-362.

Nickel, P., Nachreiner, F. 2003. *Sensitivity and diagnosticity of the 0.1-Hz component of heart rate variability as an indicator of mental workload.* Hum. Factors 45, 575-590.

Ohira, T., Roux, A.V., Prineas, R.J., Kizilbash, M.A., Carnethon, M.R., Folsom, A.R. 2008. *Associations of psychosocial factors with heart rate and its short-term variability: multi-ethnic study of atherosclerosis.* Psychosom. Med. 70, 141-146.

Ozgocmen, S., Yoldas, T., Yigiter, R., Kaya, A., Ardicoglu, O. 2006. *R-R interval variation and sympathetic skin response in fibromyalgia.* Arch. Med. Res. 37,630-634.

Pan, J. & Tompkins, W.J. *"A Real-Time QRS Detection Algorithm", IEEE Transactions on Biomedical Engineering Vol BME-32 No. 3,* March 1985.

Pattyn, N., Neyt, X., Henderickx, D, Soetens, E. 2008. *Psychophysiological investigation of vigilance decrement: boredom or cognitive fatigue?* Physiol. Behav. 93, 369-378.

Penninx, B.W., Beekman, A.T.F., Honig, A., Deeg, D.J.H., Schoever, R.A., van Eijk, J.T.M., Tilburg, W. 2001. *Depression and cardiac mortality: results from community based longitudinal study.* Arch. Gen. Psychiatry 58, 221–227.

Pieper, S., Brosschot, J.F. 2005. *Prolonged stress-related cardiovascular activation: Is there any?* Ann. Behav. Med. 30, 91-103.

Pieper, S., Brosschot, J.F., van der Leeden, R., Thayer, J.F. 2007. *Cardiac effects of momentary assessed worry episodes and stressful events.* Psychosom. Med. 69, 901-909.

Princi, T., Accardo, A., Peterec, D. 2004. *Linear and non-linear parameters of heart rate variability during static and dynamic exercise in a high-performance dinghy sailor.* Biomed. Sci. Instrum. 40, 311-316.

Porges, S.W. 1995. *Orienting in a defensive world: Mammalian modifications of our evolutionary heritage. A polyvagal theory.* Psychophysiology, 32, 301-318.

Porges, S.W. (1997). *Emotion: An evolutionary by-product of the neural regulation of the autonomic nervous system.* In C. S. Carter, B. Kirkpatrick, & I.I.

Lederhendler (eds.), *The Integrative Neurobiology of Affiliation,* Annals of the New York Academy of Sciences, 807, 62-77.

Porges, S.W., Doussard-Roosevelt, J.A., Stifter, C.A., McClenny, B.D., Riniolo, T.C. (1999). *Sleep state and vagal regulation of heart period patterns in the human newborn: An extension of the polyvagal theory.* Psychophysiology, 36(1), 14-21.

Rush, A.J., George, M.S., Sackeim, H.A., Marangell, L.B., Husain, M.M., Giller, C., Nahas, Z., Haines, S., Simpson, R.K., Goodman, R. 2000. *Vagus Nerve Stimulation (VNS) for Treatment-Resistant Depressions: A Multicenter Study.* Biological Psychiatry, 47, 276-286.

Ryan, M., Gevirtz, R. 2004. *Biofeedback based psychophysiological treatment in a primary care setting: An initial feasibility study.* Appl. Psychophysiol. Biofeedback 29(2), 79-93.

Siepmann, M., Aykac, V., Unterdörfer, J., Petrowski, K., Mueck-Weymann, M. 2008. *Pilot Study on the Effects of Heart Rate Variability Biofeedback in Patients with Depression and in Healthy Subjects.* Applied Psychophysiology and Biofeedback 33(4), 1573-3270.

Song, H.S., Lehrer, P.M. 2003. *The effects of specific respiratory rates on heart rate and heart rate variability.* Appl Psychophysiol Biofeedback. 28(1), 13-2.

Strack, B. W. 2003. *Effect of heart rate variability (HRV) biofeedback on batting performance in baseball* (Doctoral dissertation ATT # 3083450) California School of Professional Psychology at Alliant International University San Diego.

Task Force of the European Society of Cardiology the North American Society of Pacing Electrophysiology. 1996. *Heart rate variability: standards of measurement, physiological interpretation and clinical use.* Circulation 93, 1043–1065.

Thayer, J.F., Friedman, B.H., Borkovec, T.D. 1996. *Autonomic characteristics of generalized anxiety disorder and worry.* Biol. Psychiatry 39, 255-266.

Thayer J., Lane, R.D. 2000. A *model of neurovisceral integration in emotion regulation and dysregulation.* J. Affective Dis. 61, 201-216.

Tucker, P., Adamson, P., Miranda, R. Jr, Scarborough, A., Williams, D., Groff, J., McLean, H. 1997. *Paroxetine increases heart rate variability in panic disorder.* J Clin Psychopharmacol, 17, 370-376.

Tulen, J.H., Bruijn, J.A., de Man, K.J., Pepplinkhuizen, L., van den Meiracker, A.H., Man in 't Veld, A.J. 1996. *Cardiovascular variability in major depressive disorder and effects of imipramine or mirtazapine.* J. Clin. Psychopharmacol. 16(20), 135-145.

Udupa, K., Sathyaprabha, T.N., Thirthalli, J., Kishore, K.R., Lavekar, G.S., Raju, T.R., & Gangadhar, B.N. 2007. *Alteration of cardiac autonomic functions in patients with major depression: A study using heart rate variability measures.* J. Affective Dis. 100, 137–141.

Umetani, K., Singer, D.H., McCraty, R., Atkinson, M., 1998. *Twenty-four hour time domain heart rate variability and heart rate: relations to age and gender over nine decades.* J. Am. Coll. Cardiol. 31, 593-601.

Vaccarino, V., Lampert, R., Bremner, J.D., Lee, F., Su, S., Maisano, C., Murrah, N.V., Jones, L., Jawed, F., Afzal, N., Ashraf, A., Goldberg, J. 2008.

Depressive symptoms and heart rate variability: evidence for a shared genetic substrate in a study of twins. Psychosom. Med. 70, 628-636.

Van Zyl, L.T., Hasegawa, T., & Nagata, K. 2008. *Effects of antidepressant treatment on heart rate variability in major depression: A quantitative review.* BioPsychoSocial Medicine, 2, 1-10.

Vaschillo, E., Lehrer, P., Rishe, N., & Konstantinov, M. (2002). *Heart rate variability biofeedback as a method for assessing baroreflex function: a preliminary study of resonance in the cardiovascular system.* Appl. Psychophysiol. Biofeedback, 27, 1–27.

Vaschillo, E.G., Vaschillo, B., Lehrer, P.M. 2006. *Characteristics of Resonance in Heart Rate Variability Stimulated by Biofeedback.* Appl. Psychophysiol. Biofeedback 29(2), 31(2), 129-142.

Wittling, W., Block, A., Genzel, S., Schweiger, E. 1998. *Hemisphere asymmetry in parasympathetic control of the heart.* Neuropsychologia 36, 461-468.

Wong, S.W., Masse, N., Kimmerly, D.S., Menon, R., Shoemaker, J.K. 2007. *Ventral medial prefrontal cortex and cardiovagal control in conscious humans.* Neuroimage. 35, 698-708.

Zanstra, Y.J., Schellekens, J.M., Schaap, C., Kooistra, L. 2006. *Vagal and sympathetic activity in burnouts during a mentally demanding workday.* Psychosom. Med. 68, 583-590.

Other Great Titles by Heart Space Publications

Dance of Light: a new way of understanding the Earth and all life forms.

All is One : an extra ordinary book that teaches difficult concepts in a simple way!

Yogi, the Tails and Teachings of a Suburban Alpha Doggy: a delightful read illustrating the wisdom and humour that animals bring to our lives.

Second Chance, Regain your Health with Tissue Salts: this book will help the full spectrum of users, from concerned parents, experienced pharmacists and health care workers.

The Art of Walking: a treasure trove of knowledge, practical guidance and inspiration in lyrical prose.

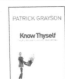

Know Thyself: a workbook that can become a lifeline for alife that works.

Towards a Soulful Sexuality: an intelligent, thought provoking and candid new perspective of sex, age and menopause for all women.

How to Write - Right!: with this book you will become the writer you have always wanted to be.

Trees, the Guardian of the Soul: a book of short stories that imparts the wisdom of the ages, appealing to all age groups.

The Halo and the Noose: a great piece of work which stimulates one to look at life differently.

Hillhairyass Poems: poems and illustrations created to entertain and support young adults.

Guided! How to Communicate with your Spirit Guides: Discover your soul's purpose and learn techniques to communicate with your spirit guides.

The Irritable Woman's Cookbook: "cooking is like sex; you have to be in the mood", says the humorous author of this Jewish cookbook.

Seasons of Our Lives: George Kouloukis shows that the alternating trends of our lives - going from good to bad and vice versa, are according to specific patterns.

The Path of Cosmic Consciousness: journey through initiation to enlightenment in the sacred Andean tradition.

What if: an encounter of simple truth about life and spirituality.

Paws and Listen to the Voices of the Animals: Read this book, then open your heart, free your mind and listen to the ancient wisdom of the animals that you love.

Spunky: Join me on my journey of becoming a cancer survivor, and against all odds a provincial badminton player.

Bleeding Heart: Bleeding Heart is a timeless fable about living life with passion. It will bring joy to your soul as you turn the pages ever faster.

Heart Space Publications
Australia: +61 450 260 348
South Africa: +27 11 431 1274
pat@heartspacebooks.com
www.heartspacebooks.com